29

[…] RISK
[…] RIES

Microbial safety of lipid-based ready-to-use foods for management of moderate acute malnutrition and severe acute malnutrition

SECOND REPORT

Food and Agriculture Organization of the United Nations
World Health Organization

Rome, 2021

Required citation:
FAO and WHO. 2021. *Microbial safety of lipid-based ready-to-use foods for management of moderate acute malnutrition and severe acute malnutrition* – Second report. Microbiological Risk Assessment Series No. 29. Rome. https://doi.org/10.4060/cb3223en

ISSN 1726-5274 [Print]
ISSN 1728-0605 [Online]
FAO ISBN 978-92-5-133930-5
WHO ISBN 978-92-4-001991-1 (print version)
WHO ISBN 978-92-4-001990-4 (electronic version)

Contents

Preface vii

Acknowledgements viii

Contributors ix

Declarations of interest xi

Abbreviations and acronyms xii

Executive summary xiii

1 Background 1

2 Introduction 4

2.1 Definitions of acute malnutrition 4

2.2 Management of MAM and SAM 5

2.3 Ready-to-use foods for acute malnutrition 6

2.3.1 Lipid-based RUF ingredients 7

2.3.2 Manufacture of RUFs for acute malnutrition 7

2.4 Relationship between malnutrition and infection 8

3 Risk assessment for lipid-based RUFs used to manage MAM and SAM 11

3.1 Hazard identification 11

3.2 Hazard characterization 17

3.3 Exposure assessment 25

3.4 Risk characterization 27

4 Managing the risk of salmonellosis from lipid-based RUFs fed to children 6–59 months of age with MAM and SAM 31

4.1 Risk-based food safety management 31

4.1.1 Good hygienic practices 31

4.1.2 Raw ingredients 32

4.1.3 Intervention technologies 32

4.1.4 Re-contamination 32

4.2 The role of microbiological testing in food safety management 33

4.2.1 Setting a microbiological criterion 38

4.2.2 Example approaches to setting a microbiological criterion for ready-to-use foods 39

5 Conclusions 45

5.1 Pathogen(s) of concern 45

5.2 Susceptibility of children with SAM relative to children of the same age without malnutrition 45

5.3 Assessing the probability of foodborne infection from RUFs 46

5.4 Potential to implement kill steps to further reduce microbial contamination 47

5.5 Microbiological criteria appropriate to lipid-based RUFs and how they should be used 48

6 Recommendations 49

6.1 Recommendations for manufacturers 49

6.2 Recommendations for agencies 51

References 53

ANNEXES

Annex 1 Overview of ready-to-use foods for acute malnutrition 68

Annex 2 Analysis of published models for dose-response of *Salmonella* and additional relevant data, including derivation of exponential dose-response models from *Salmonella* outbreaks associated with low-moisture foods 74

Annex 3 Re-analysis of Teunis *et al.* (2010) dataset as a beta-Poisson model and comparison with the FAO/WHO (2002) *Salmonella* dose-response model 77

TABLES

Table 1	Pathogens identified as causes of serious infections in South African children with severe acute malnutrition	12
Table 2	Pathogenic micro-organisms considered in the hazard identification	15
Table 3	Examples of the predicted risk of gastrointestinal salmonellosis for SAM children receiving a full course of RUFs (62 servings) based on different levels and frequencies of RUF contamination	28
Table 4:	Relationship between the number of 100 g servings analysed and the probability of accepting a contaminated lot	29

FIGURES

Figure 1.	Community management of acute malnutrition (CMAM) is the most widely accepted model for managing malnutrition, and uses triage for management options for acute malnutrition	5
Figure 2.	Generalized production flow diagram for lipid-based RUFs	8
Figure 3	Examples of relationships between dose and probability of gastrointestinal non-typhoidal Salmonella infection	19
Figure 4	Examples of the predicted relationships between dose and probability of gastrointestinal non-typhoidal Salmonella infection from different models	20
Figure 5	Examples of the predicted relationships between dose and probability of gastrointestinal non-typhoidal Salmonella infection from different models with both modelled responses shown on a linear scale	21
Figure 6	FAO and WHO (2002) "dose-vs-probability of gastrointestinal non-typhoidal salmonellosis" model	22
Figure 7	FAO/WHO (2002) “dose-vs-probability of gastrointestinal non-typhoidal salmonellosis” model compared with a beta-Poisson model fitted to the expanded salmonellosis database (after correction for transcription errors) presented in Teunis *et al.* (2010)	24
Figure 8	The relative sensitivity of different sampling plans to detect contamination of RUF meals by different levels of *Salmonella* and their relationship to realistic contamination levels.	35

Preface

This was the second meeting to address the issue of microbial safety of lipid-based ready-to-use foods for management of moderate and severe acute malnutrition. The deliberations of this meeting served to build on the findings of the first meeting, and to revise and update the recommendations of that meeting according to new information generated in the meantime. The first meeting was implemented in a crisis situation where there was an urgent need to address the microbiological safety of these products, and the recommendations from that meeting reflect that situation and were, as a result, more reactive in nature. This second meeting was able to take a more holistic view of the microbiological safety of these products and look towards a more long-term approach to managing the safety of these products in a proactive and sustainable manner.

Acknowledgements

FAO and WHO would like to express their appreciation to all those who contributed to the preparation of this report through their participation in the expert meeting that was held on 8–11 December 2014, and the follow-up discussions in 2015, for their time, expertise, data and other relevant information. Appreciation is extended to the manufacturers of lipid-based ready-to-use foods for the management of moderate and severe acute malnutrition that shared microbiological data from their monitoring programmes as well as other relevant information with the expert meeting. FAO and WHO are also grateful to Médecins Sans Frontières, the United Nations Children's Fund, and the World Food Programme for the data that they shared from their monitoring and auditing programmes, which greatly facilitated an understanding of the product and its production.

Particular appreciation is extended to Morris Potter, who liaised with all the relevant parties and provided technical oversight to the development and completion of the report.

Contributors

EXPERTS

Larry Beuchat, University of Georgia, United States of America

Robert Buchanan, University of Maryland, United States of America

Seamus Fanning, University College Dublin, Ireland

Stephen Forsythe, Nottingham Trent University, United Kingdom of Great Britain and Northern Ireland

Henrik Friis, University of Copenhagen, Denmark

Mark Manary, Washington University, United States of America

Peter McClure, Mondelēz International, United Kingdom of Great Britain and Northern Ireland

Tom Ross, University of Tasmania, Australia

Phillip Tarr, Washington University, United States of America

RESOURCE PERSONS

Pauline Allemand, FAO, Italy

Hanane Bouzambou, World Food Programme, Italy

Odile Caron, Médecins Sans Frontières, Switzerland

Darrell Donahue, Michigan State University, United States of America

Alison Fleet, United Nations Children's Fund, United States of America

Kerstin Hanson, Médecins Sans Frontières, Switzerland

Peter Jakobsen, United Nations Children's Fund, United States of America

Charles Jelensperger, World Food Programme, Italy

Jan Komrska, United Nations Children's Fund, United States of America

Lynnda Kriess, World Food Programme, Italy

Catherine Leclercq, FAO, Italy

Rufino Perez, United States Agency for International Development, United States of America

Shane Prigge, World Food Programme, Italy

Jolanta Wozniak, United Nations Children's Fund, United States of America

Marcel Zwietering, Wageningen University, The Netherlands

SECRETARIAT

Peter Karim Ben Embarek, WHO, Switzerland

Sarah Cahill, FAO, Italy

Morris Potter, FAO, Italy

Kang Zhou, FAO, Italy

Jeffrey LeJeune, FAO, Italy

Satoko Murakami, WHO, Switzerland

Haruka Igarashi, WHO, Switzerland

Declaration of interest

All participants completed a declaration of interest form in advance of the meeting. Four of the experts indicated interests in their declarations:

- Peter McClure works in the private sector, and noted that his previous employer had an interest in developing products for malnourished children. This interest ended when he changed employment in April 2014.
- Mark Manary noted that he had founded a not-for-profit organization that advocated for the treatment of severely malnourished children and in doing so used ready-to-use therapeutic foods. However, he had no financial interests in this.
- Henrik Friis indicated that his research group had received resources from the private sector, including from producers of ready-to-use foods to undertake nutrition-related studies.
- Stephen Forsythe works in academia, and noted that his research was partially funded by the private sector.

All of the declarations, together with any updates, were made known and available to all the participants at the beginning of the meeting. Owing to the focus of the meeting on the safety aspects of the products under discussion, rather than their value in the management of moderate and severe acute malnutrition, all experts participated fully in the meeting. All the experts participated in their individual capacity and not as representatives of their country, government or organization.

Abbreviations and acronyms

ALOP	appropriate level of protection
Aw	water activity
CFU	colony-forming unit
CMAM	community management of acute malnutrition
D value	decimal reduction time
EB	Enterobacteriaceae
GHP	good hygienic practice
GMP	good manufacturing practice
HACCP	Hazard Analysis and Critical Control Point (System)
ICMSF	International Commission on Microbiological Specifications for Foods
ID50	dose of an infectious organism required to produce infection in 50 percent of the experimental subjects
LBT	lot-based testing
LMF	low-moisture food
LNS	lipid-based nutrient supplements
MAM	moderate acute malnutrition
MC	microbiological criterion/criteria
MSF	Médecins Sans Frontières
MUAC	mid-upper arm circumference
PCV	process control verification
PRP	prerequisite programmes
RUF	ready-to-use food
RUSF	ready-to-use supplementary food
RUTF	ready-to-use therapeutic food
SAM	severe acute malnutrition
UNICEF	United Nations Children's Fund
UTI	urinary tract infection
WFP	World Food Programme

Executive summary

Lipid-based ready-to-use foods (RUFs) for the nutritional management of moderate acute malnutrition (MAM) and severe acute malnutrition (SAM) are provided to children from 6 months to 59 months of age within the context of emergency feeding programmes supervised by governments, Médecins Sans Frontières (MSF), the United Nations Children's Fund (UNICEF), the World Food Programme (WFP), and other non-governmental organizations. The FAO/WHO expert meeting held in December 2014 considered microbial contamination of lipid-based RUFs and the risk of foodborne infections in the malnourished population of children that consume RUFs. The goals of the expert meeting were to: review the status of the microbiological safety of lipid-based RUFs used to manage MAM and SAM; conduct a comprehensive risk assessment; provide guidance to producers on the general approach and requirements for manufacturing RUFs that are safe for their intended use; and provide guidance to the agencies that purchase RUFs on how best to judge their microbiological safety.

Ready-to-use foods consist of powdered or ground ingredients embedded in a lipid- or protein-based matrix, resulting in an energy- and nutrition-dense food. An RUF is typically a lipid-rich paste, made from ground peanuts (*Arachis hypogaea*), milk products, sugar, oil and a pre-mix containing vitamins and minerals. The RUF manufacturing process involves receiving raw materials, appropriate mixing, intermediate treatment (heating and grinding) and the filling of sachets. Some manufacturers have added thermal processing as an additional control step for pathogenic bacteria. Lipid-based RUFs have low levels of biologically available water and, therefore, share the microbiological and food safety characteristics of other low-moisture foods.

In conducting the hazard identification part of the risk assessment, the expert committee reviewed: evidence of anatomical and physiological derangement associated with malnutrition that could influence susceptibility to infections; data on bacterial, viral and parasitic infections identified in malnourished children; and data on foodborne infections that have been associated with low-moisture foods. Based on this review, the expert committee considered that children with SAM have an increase in susceptibility to bacteraemia and sepsis that is probably between twofold and fivefold compared with children who are not malnourished and are of the same age and live in the same communities. While some of the infections commonly identified in malnourished children can sometimes be foodborne, the expert committee could find no evidence that any of the infections reported in the medical literature were foodborne or were associated with lipid-based RUFs.

On the basis of its common occurrence as a cause of infections and serious illnesses in children with SAM, and its documented ability to contaminate, survive in, and cause outbreaks of illness associated with low-moisture foods similar to RUFs, the expert committee concluded that *Salmonella* is the pathogen of most concern in lipid-based RUFs. Although Salmonella can survive for many months in low-moisture foods such as RUFs (slowly dying off at a rate determined by the storage temperature), *Salmonella* cannot grow in these foods. Qualitative testing for *Salmonella* in RUFs since 2012 has demonstrated that approximately five 25-g samples in every 1 000 (0.5 percent prevalence) contained *Salmonella*. This suggests that approximately 1 in every 200 sachets of about 100 g each will contain one or more *Salmonella* cells, approximately 1 in 30 000 000 sachets will contain 10 or more cells, and approximately 1 in 10^{13} sachets will contain 1 000 or more cells of *Salmonella*.

Many outbreaks of foodborne salmonellosis have been determined to be associated with low-moisture foods that were contaminated at low levels. Therefore, the expert committee carefully considered the qualitative microbiological analyses of RUFs and the contamination levels that could be inferred, and entered into an extended deliberation of dose-response modelling to find a path toward a reasonable approximation of the likely morbidity and mortality in SAM children that could be anticipated from consumption of RUFs contaminated at the estimated levels and observed frequency. The expert committee found that the FAO/WHO (2002) dose-response model for foodborne salmonellosis was its most defensible model option and, adjusting the model to accommodate for the increased susceptibility of children with SAM, estimated the incidence of gastrointestinal salmonellosis likely to result from a range of cumulative exposure doses during a 31-day exposure window in order to guide safety standard setting by the agencies that purchase RUFs for use in malnourished populations.

Consistently producing RUFs at an acceptable level of safety requires active control of the entire process, including maintenance of good hygienic practices, raw-ingredient sourcing controls, use of appropriate intervention technologies, and prevention of re-contamination. The report elaborates general guidance in these four areas to help direct facility- and product-specific process-control planning and operations.

The expert committee determined that sampling and microbiological testing (for pathogens and indicator organisms) of food ingredients, the food processing environment, and food products are effective tools for verifying compliance with preventive and sanitation programmes, process control and sanitary conditions, Hazard Analysis and Critical Control Point (HACCP)-based systems, and microbiological criteria. However, the expert committee found that sampling and testing finished products are inefficient and ineffective means to guarantee food safety. Nonetheless, for products from manufacturers without a history of production to adequate levels of safety, or that operate with the principles of good hygiene only but without preventive controls and intervention technologies, the expert committee found few alternatives to rigorous monitoring of ingredients and the production environment, plus end-product testing for lot release. Under these conditions of possibly wide variation in contamination levels, sampling would be appropriate at greater intensity than would otherwise be justified by the modest (i.e. less than fivefold) increase in susceptibility of the intended consumers. The safety of RUFs can be demonstrated for manufacturers with a history of safety compliance, documented process control, and validated intervention technologies by monitoring the process in real time with physical or chemical tests to verify that the process is operating as designed, plus additional periodic microbiological testing (primarily with indicator organisms) to verify that the food safety system is under control, rather than lot-by-lot testing. It should be the goal of agencies using RUFs to move all manufacturers into this category of production.

Finally, the expert committee described three approaches that purchasers of RUFs might use to establish microbiological criteria to assure the safety of RUFs and to communicate to manufacturers their safety expectations. These approaches are: (i) reference to existing standards established for similar low-moisture foods; (ii) determining an acceptable increase in risk over the pre-existing baseline of illness from other sources of exposure; and (iii) process verification sampling using the moving window technique. The microbiological criteria derived by each of these approaches accomplish different purposes, and which is most appropriate is determined by the conditions of manufacture and use.

1

Background

Lipid-based ready-to-use foods (RUFs) for the nutritional management of moderate acute malnutrition (MAM) and severe acute malnutrition (SAM) can be life-saving. They are provided to children from 6 months to 59 months of age within the context of emergency feeding programmes supervised by governments, Médecins Sans Frontières (MSF), the United Nations Children's Fund (UNICEF), the World Food Programme (WFP), and other non-governmental organizations.

This FAO/WHO expert meeting, held in December 2014, considered microbial contamination of lipid-based RUFs. The intent was to be comprehensive in scope, but to focus recommendations on guiding food producers and agencies that distribute lipid-based RUFs so that the risk to malnourished children of foodborne infections would be reduced to the extent practically possible. All types of microbial contamination were considered, encompassing viruses, bacteria, fungi and parasites. The agenda addressed food safety issues similar to those discussed in December 2012 by another FAO/WHO expert committee, but the context then had been more focused on the risk associated with *Cronobacter* in these products and how to manage an ongoing and urgent issue of contamination with *Cronobacter* spp., as elaborated below.

In 2012, UNICEF and the WFP found, in certain lots of RUFs, bacterial species of the genus *Cronobacter*, which have been documented as causing foodborne infections in young infants (Forsythe, Dickins and Jolley, 2014; Holy and Forsythe, 2014). They requested the assistance of FAO and WHO to determine the clinical significance of foodborne exposure of the intended consumers to *Cronobacter* species at the levels of contamination identified, and for general guidance on the microbial purchase specifications used when obtaining RUFs from producers. Therefore, FAO and WHO convened a technical meeting at FAO headquarters, Rome, Italy, on 11–14 December 2012, to address these issues (FAO and WHO, 2016a). The 2012 expert committee reviewed the information provided by the WFP, UNICEF and MSF, and published data on infections in the population of interest and the microbial contamination of low-moisture foods (LMFs), the general food category that includes lipid-based RUFs. After conducting a risk assessment based on available information, the experts concluded that *Salmonella* was the pathogen of greatest concern for these products, and that its control should be the focus of efforts to ensure the safety of these products. Considering the Codex Principles and Guidelines for the Establishment and Application of Microbiological Criteria Related to Foods (CAC, 1997), which highlight the importance of demonstrating the need to establish a microbiological criterion (MC), it was considered relevant to establish such a criterion for *Salmonella* in RUFs, but that there was not adequate justification at that point to establish such a criterion for other pathogens, such as *Cronobacter*. The 2012 expert committee expressed concern about the level of ingredient and process control demonstrated by producers of lipid-based RUFs, and provided guidance on sanitation and other prerequisite programmes (PRPs), good manufacturing practices (GMPs), good hygienic practices (GHPs), Hazard Analysis and Critical Control Point (HACCP) and sampling strategies that would provide greater assurance of process control and product safety. The 2012 expert committee also encouraged research on manufacturing processes that would deliver an adequate reduction in pathogen numbers. The 2012 expert committee requested additional end-product microbiological data and, based on those results, recommended interim end-product purchase specifications for *Salmonella* and for Enterobacteriaceae (EB), a family of Gram-negative bacteria commonly used by the food industry to indicate the level of hygiene. The goals of the recommendations were to achieve sufficiently low levels of bacterial density in RUFs to protect the intended consumers, and to drive continuous improvement in production practices and conditions, with specifications that were generally achievable, in order to assure the availability of an uninterrupted supply of lipid-based RUFs.

The 2012 expert committee further recommended (FAO and WHO, 2016a) that WHO and FAO enlist another group of experts after two years to: re-visit the issue of the microbial safety of lipid-based RUFs; conduct another risk assessment based on the accrued microbiological data on the product, newly published reports on immunology and infectious diseases in malnourished populations, and additional information on LMFs; and revise the recommendations for purchase specifications. Therefore, FAO and WHO convened a new technical meeting on 8–11 December 2014 at FAO headquarters in Rome, with the following goals:

- Review the status of the microbiological safety of lipid-based RUFs used to manage MAM and SAM.

- Review and update the risk assessment.
- Provide further guidance to producers on the general approach and requirements for manufacturing LMFs that are safe for their intended use, and aspects of PRPs, GMPs, GHPs, programmes of process control assurance, and HACCP programmes used by other parts of the food industry that manufacture LMFs.
- Review and possibly revise the guidance and recommendations to the agencies that purchase lipid-based RUFs on how to best judge their microbial safety.

2

Introduction

The prevalence of acute malnutrition (wasting) in children under 5 years of age was estimated to be approximately 8 percent globally in 2013, out of which almost one-third was SAM (UNICEF, WHO and World Bank, 2015). Therefore, approximately 51 million children under 5 years are acutely wasted, and 17 million of these children are severely wasted. Approximately 3 million childhood deaths annually are attributable to acute malnutrition. In addition, there are significant cognitive and economic consequences of malnutrition for those who survive. When acute malnutrition is layered on chronic malnutrition, the clinical consequences are more severe. Acute malnutrition results from poor feeding practices, illness and inadequate food intake, and possibly other exogenous factors. Diets that are inadequate in terms of quantity and quality result in energy, protein, lipid and micronutrient deficiencies, and each deficiency is linked to specific complications. Acute malnutrition is often seen in conjunction with other health problems, such as recurrent infections, particularly malaria, respiratory illness, and diarrhoea (Picot *et al.*, 2012; Manary, personal communication, December 2014). Both MAM and SAM are associated with increased severity of common infectious diseases, and the accompanying mortality is almost always the result of infection (WHO, UNICEF, SCN and UNICEF, 2007). Given this potentially increased susceptibility to infection with specific pathogens, rapidly correcting the nutritional status of the children is an urgent medical necessity, and the provision of products that carry a low risk of microbiological contamination is seen as a priority.

2.1 DEFINITIONS OF ACUTE MALNUTRITION

Severe acute malnutrition (SAM) is diagnosed when a child's weight-for-height index is less than three standard deviations below the median of the WHO growth standard, and/or the mid-upper arm circumference (MUAC) is less than 115 mm, and/or the child has nutritional oedema. Moderate acute malnutrition (MAM) is diagnosed when a child's weight-for-height index is between two and three standard deviations below the median of the WHO growth standard, and/or the MUAC is less than 125 mm, but above or equal to 115 mm (WHO, 2012).

2.2 MANAGEMENT OF MAM AND SAM

Community management of acute malnutrition (CMAM) is the most widely accepted model for managing malnutrition, and it was used in 61 countries in 2013. This model triages children into categories of care (Figure 1):

- inpatient therapeutic care of complicated SAM;
- outpatient therapeutic care of uncomplicated SAM;
- supplementary feeding to correct MAM.

The model includes community mobilization and outreach to encourage and support early detection and enrolment of children with acute malnutrition. This approach has improved programme coverage over programmes that depend solely on inpatient care, but many children are still not reached.

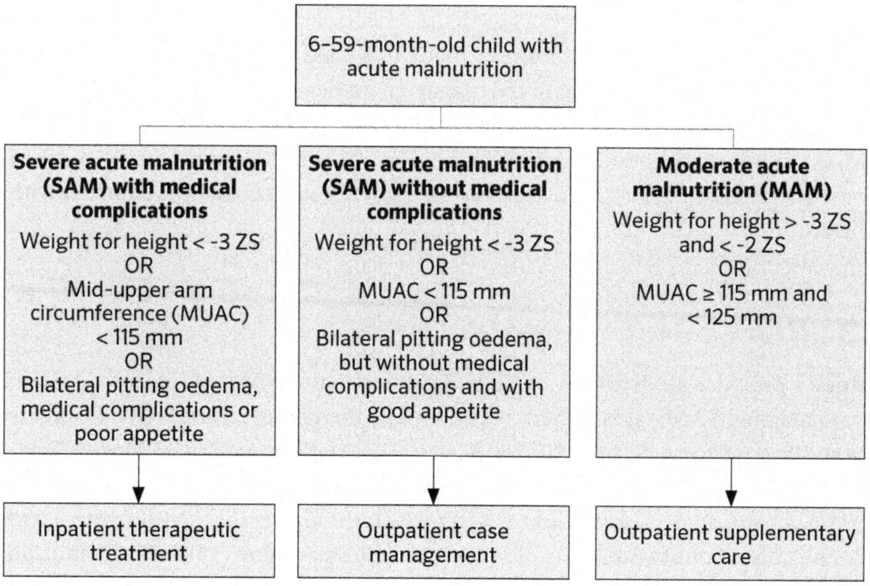

FIGURE 1. Community management of acute malnutrition (CMAM) is the most widely accepted model for managing malnutrition, and uses triage for management options for acute malnutrition

As part of CMAM, specifically trained healthcare workers at community-based health centres provide care to acutely malnourished children and their mothers. Malnourished children with medical complications or oedema are managed as inpatients within the centre until their health situation is stabilized. Children who have appetite and do not have medical complications are managed through outpatient services. International protocols outline the treatment standards for the three categories. Nutritional management includes a provision of specialized nutritional products in the form of RUFs for the child to consume at home, along with instructions about feeding and good hygiene (Annan, Webb and Brown, 2014). In addition, a number of other health services are provided, including routine medicines and nutrition counselling. In the last decade, CMAM programmes have been scaled up significantly, with 61 countries using some form of CMAM now, compared with only 9 countries in 2005 (Gray *et al.*, 2014). Community management of acute malnutrition is part of a larger community-based, multisectoral health and nutrition package to prevent illness and undernutrition. Guidance is provided on how to consume the products, how to keep the food between uses, and how to continue to breastfeed and provide potable drinking water.

Children in treatment programmes are followed weekly, twice monthly or monthly depending on the specific context. Monitoring is conducted on the individual child to ensure that children are treated appropriately and effectively, which helps to continually improve the services.

UNICEF and the WFP, in addition to many other aid agencies, procure RUFs to support CMAM programming in the management of acute malnutrition. UNICEF and the WFP are, along with WHO, the lead United Nations agencies providing CMAM support to national governments. In 2012, these programmes resulted in the treatment of 2.6 million children with SAM and 4.6 million children with MAM.

2.3 READY-TO-USE FOODS FOR ACUTE MALNUTRITION

Annex 1 provides an overview of RUFs for acute malnutrition. Lipid-based RUFs for managing SAM, also called ready-to-use therapeutic foods (RUTFs), are energy- and nutrient-dense (520–550 kcal/100 g). Management of SAM with lipid-based RUFs requires daily provision of 100–135 kcal/kg for 6–10 weeks, until the child has gained adequate weight (WHO, 2013a). On average, a child with SAM can consume about two sachets of lipid-based RUFs per day (1 000 kcal), and can achieve sufficient nutrient intake for complete recovery. While lipid-based RUFs for management of SAM must be served with potable water, no other foods besides breast milk are necessary to rehabilitate a severely malnourished child.

Lipid-based RUFs for the management of MAM, also called ready-to-use supplementary food (RUSFs), are a type of RUF specifically designed for the management of MAM in children 6–59 months of age. For the management of MAM, 92–100 g of lipid-based RUFs, with an energy density of 513–550 kcal/100 g, are recommended as a daily ration. This ration is consumed by the child in addition to breast milk and other family foods for about 2–3 months (WHO, 2013a).

2.3.1 Lipid-based RUF ingredients

Ready-to-use foods consist of powdered or ground ingredients embedded in a lipid- or protein-based matrix, resulting in an energy- and nutrition-dense food. They are typically produced in the form of a lipid-rich paste, made from ground peanuts (usually *Arachis hypogaea*, more correctly called groundnuts), milk products, sugar, oil and a pre-mix containing vitamins and minerals. They can also include legumes such as soybeans and chickpeas, and cereal flours such as rice, millet, oats and wheat.

As the name implies, RUFs do not need preparation before consumption, increasing their practicality where cooking fuel and facilities are limited. These foods are given to children from the caregiver's finger to the child's mouth, or are eaten by the child directly from the sachet. Lipid-based RUFs have a water activity (A_w) of < 0.5, thus eliminating the risk of microbial growth. They have a shelf life of about 24 months (WHO, UNICEF, SCN and UNICEF, 2007).

Other lipid-based nutrient supplement (LNS) products are used in CMAM programmes, including medium-quantity LNS, large-quantity LNS and small-quantity LNS. These products are not used to manage acute malnutrition, but rather are used as supplements to prevent malnutrition and boost nutritional content of staple family foods. These products are not the subject of this report.

2.3.2 Manufacture of RUFs for acute malnutrition

The RUF manufacturing process involves receiving raw materials, appropriate mixing, intermediate treatment (heating and grinding), and the filling of sachets (Figure 2). Some manufacturers have added thermal processing as an additional control step for pathogenic bacteria, including *Salmonella*.

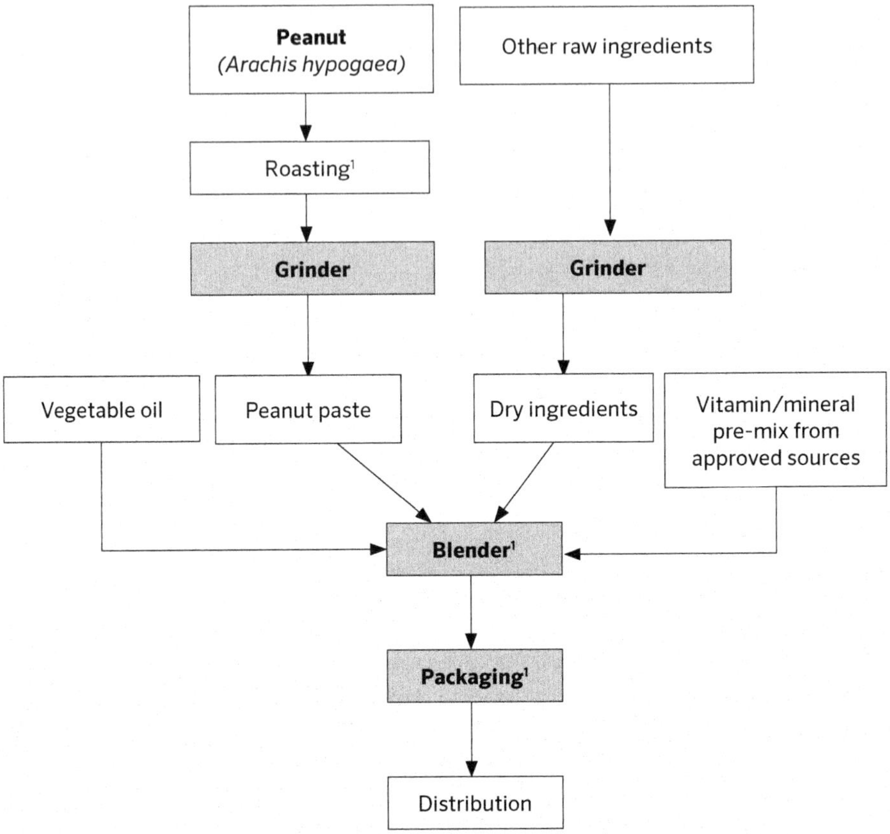

FIGURE 2. Generalized production flow diagram for lipid-based RUFs

[1] There are at least three possible points in the production flow where heat could be applied, i.e. roasting before grinding; heating after blending; and heating post-packaging. Currently, the only heat step that could be effectively implemented in all production settings is roasting. Research is still under way on the potential application of heat at other steps in the process.

Salmonella cannot grow in LMFs owing to the low water activity, although the ability of *Salmonella* to persist in dry foods for long periods of time is well documented (see Section 3.3).

2.4 RELATIONSHIP BETWEEN MALNUTRITION AND INFECTION

Children in low-income countries are almost universally breastfed, but are rarely exclusively breastfed to the age of six months as recommended. Hence, low-quality, plant-based, complementary foods are introduced prematurely or inappropriately, and soon thereafter children receive a family diet with low nutrient and energy density, and usually devoid of animal-source foods. Because of the early introduction of complementary foods, as well as crowding, contaminated water, poor sanitation and hygiene, and geophagy (the practice of eating soil), young children are repeatedly exposed to a diversity of pathogens (bacterial, viral, protozoan and helminths), causing frequent and recurrent infections that may become latent and chronic. As outlined in the literature review below, undernutrition generally increases the likelihood and severity of such infections. The resulting inflammation and superimposed focal lesions and lethargy further impair nutrient intake and absorption, and ultimately nutritional status, thus producing a vicious cycle, leading to stunting and/or wasting.

Considering all indicators of undernutrition, including low birth weight, stunting and micronutrient malnutrition, undernutrition afflicts hundreds of millions of children worldwide and plays a role in almost half of childhood deaths (Black *et al.*, 2008). The most common contributors to undernutrition are inadequate dietary intake, infections and poverty. Food-based interventions that include ready-to-use, low-moisture, lipid-based pastes often are employed to prevent or limit the consequences of acute malnutrition.

Children with MAM are at increased risk of SAM, and even with MAM are roughly three times more likely to die from common communicable diseases than if they were not malnourished (Black *et al.*, 2008; Fernandez, Himes and De Onis, 2001). Worldwide, MAM and SAM together cause approximately 11.5 percent of total deaths of children under 5 years of age (Black *et al.*, 2013).

A substantial amount of epidemiological evidence indicates that low weight for height, weight for length and MUAC are strongly associated with a 5–20-fold increased risk of mortality (WHO, 2013a). Indeed, SAM is such an important risk factor for bacteraemia (i.e. the presence of bacteria in the blood) that invasive bacterial disease can usually be reasonably suspected on the basis of malnutrition (Berkley *et al.*, 2005). Sepsis is a life-threatening clinical response to bacteraemia, and can manifest in a variety of ways, depending on the age and condition of the bacteraemic host.

Improving children's nutritional status enhances their ability to fight infections in general, decreasing susceptibility to infection and decreasing the severity of infections that occur. However, if the lipid-based RUF used to manage MAM and SAM is itself contaminated at a pathogen level that might cause infection, the resulting illness might exacerbate the impact of the pre-existing malnutrition the RUF is being used to address. Acute malnutrition predisposes children to more frequent and severe diarrhoea (Lima *et al.*, 1992), and the illness can, in turn, worsen malnutrition (Patwari, 1999). Thus, the relationship between acute malnutrition and diarrhoea is bidirectional, and it is essential to optimize the safety of RUFs while maximizing the number of malnourished children served.

3

Risk assessment for lipid-based RUFs used to manage MAM and SAM

3.1 HAZARD IDENTIFICATION

For the purposes of this deliberation, the expert committee defined pathogens as microbes that were highly likely to cause serious illness in children. Their presence in blood, urine or cerebrospinal fluid (i.e. sites that are normally free of such micro-organisms in a person who is clinically well) substantiate their pathogenic roles. Limited gastrointestinal infections (i.e. those without extra-intestinal microbial dissemination) cannot be easily aetiologically defined or attributed to a food source, as children in these venues often have one or more such pathogens in their stools when they do not have diarrhoea (Page *et al.*, 2013). During the consultation, opinions were rendered as to the likelihood that severely malnourished children are at increased risk of serious bacterial infections. The discussions also included potentially foodborne viruses, based on the frequency with which they cause infection and the plausibility of their transmission via foods.

Documented bacteraemia and serious bacterial infection in children with SAM occur more frequently than in children without malnutrition living in the same environment. A systematic review of bacteraemia in South African children with SAM included 3 766 cultures, of which 21 percent yielded a pathogen. The rates of bacteraemia in 900 hospitalized children with SAM and 4 497 who were not malnourished were 8.3 percent and 4.8 percent, respectively (Berkowitz, 1984). This study was conducted in an era when all children with SAM were hospitalized (Table 1). The greatest disparity in bacteraemia rates was seen in Malawi: 4.8 percent in 1 388 children without SAM, and 20.6 percent in 703 children with SAM (Bronzan *et al.*, 2007).

TABLE 1. Pathogens identified as causes of serious infections in South African children with severe acute malnutrition

Most commonly identified	Non-typhoidal *Salmonella, Escherichia coli, Klebsiella pneumoniae, Streptococcus pneumoniae*
Less often identified	*Salmonella typhi, Staphylococcus aureus,* Group A beta-haemolytic *Streptococcus*
Least often identified	*Citrobacter* spp., *Enterococcus* spp., *Haemophilus influenzae*

Source: Berkowitz, 1984.

The pathophysiology of infections associated with SAM is still largely unknown. However, for working purposes, these events can be grouped into three categories – before, during and post nutritional intervention (with "nutritional intervention" representing consumption of lipid-based RUFs). The before-intervention infections are those that are evident on presentation for nutritional intervention with RUFs, and such acute episodes are often the reason for seeking attention for the malnutrition. The during-intervention infections are those that become clinically apparent after nutritional management with RUFs has commenced. The post-intervention infections are those that occur in the community, following discharge from a feeding programme. Table 1 presents the best available data regarding the aetiology of life-threatening bacterial infections in children at the time of presentation with SAM. The expert committee could not determine how many acquired infections occurred during nutritional intervention with RUFs, and which could be plausibly related to ingested RUFs. Moreover, some of these children would already have received lipid-based RUFs for MAM, further complicating attempts to identify a source. The profile of such potentially intervention-related illnesses would be those that present with a clinical deterioration (fever, diarrhoea or emesis) one or more days after RUFs have been introduced, and continuing for about a week after RUF feeding has stopped. This is the acute infection model, and such instances would be the episodes most credibly related to contaminated lipid-based RUFs. Post-discharge deaths are presumably also bacterial in origin, based on their preventability by antibiotics (Trehan *et al.*, 2013).

It is presumed that hosts in the settings of interest are at increased risk of infection because of compromised immune response or other disorders. However, the evidence for this is only modest. For example, HIV confers only a 2.6-fold greater risk of having *Salmonella* bacteraemia in Kenyan children (95 percent CI: 1.5–4.6) (Brent *et al.*, 2006). As stated above, to determine the increased risk of bacteraemia and sepsis in children with SAM compared with children who were not malnourished, the expert committee compared culture-positive rates of serious bacterial infection from several sites in sub-Saharan Africa in five studies that compared well-nourished and SAM children in the same setting (Berkowitz, 1984; Norton *et al.*, 2004; Bronzan *et al.*, 2007; Bachou *et al.*, 2006; Berkley *et al.*, 2005). The difference in risk for bacteraemia and sepsis in these two paediatric populations was 2.1–3.4, and was statistically unlikely to exceed 5.5 ($P < 0.05$, Grubbs test). The estimated difference in risk was consistent among the five studies, and *Salmonella* was among the commonly identified pathogens in each study. Considering that the likely increase in susceptibility to bacteraemia and sepsis associated with SAM was greater than twofold but less than fivefold, the expert committee settled on an estimated increase in susceptibility of 3.5-fold for the purposes of this report.

It is likely that some immune impairment that accompanies malnutrition could predispose the children to systemic or severe infections (Rytter *et al.*, 2014). Medical literature reviewed by the expert committee found evidence of the following:

- increased gut permeability (Behrens *et al.*, 1987; Brewster *et al.*, 1997; Hossain *et al.*, 2010; Boaz *et al.*, 2013; Sullivan, *et al.*, 1992);
- abnormal histology of the small bowel (Behrens *et al.*, 1987; Green and Heyworth, 1980; Theron, Wittmann and Prinsloo, 1971; Shiner, Redmond and Hansen, 1973; Stanfield, Hutt and Tunnicliffe, 1965);
- impaired secretory protective factors (Reddy, Raghuramulu and Bhaskaram, 1976; Beatty *et al.*, 1983).

However, leucocyte counts and natural killer cell (a type of cytotoxic lymphocyte that is critical to innate immunity) concentrations appear generally undiminished in SAM (Hughes *et al.*, 2009; Keusch *et al.*, 1977a, 1977b; Rosen *et al.*, 1975; Schopfer and Douglas, 1976a, 1976b; Purtilo *et al.*, 1976; Fongwo, Arinola and Salimonu, 1999; Najera *et al.*, 2001, 2004, 2007; Lotfy, Saleh and el-Barbari, 1998; Nassar *et al.*, 2007; Nassar, El-Batrawy and Nagy, 2009; Rikimaru *et al.*, 1998; Salimonu *et al.*, 1982, 1983). In addition, variability has been observed in both:

- granulocyte function (Keusch *et al.*, 1977b; Rosen *et al.*, 1975; Schopfer and Douglas, 1976a, 1976b; Purtilo *et al.*, 1976; Lotfy, Saleh and el-Barbari, 1998; Vasquez-Garibay *et al.*, 2002, 2004; Goyal *et al.*, 1981; Reddy *et al.*, 1976; Tejada *et al.*, 1964; Douglas and Schopfer, 1974; Shousha and Kamel, 1972; Carvalho Neves Forte, Martins Campos and Carneiro Leao, 1984; Chhangani *et al.*, 1985; Bhaskaram, 1980; Bhaskaram and Reddy, 1982b; Shilotri, 1976; Raman, 1992; Altay *et al.*, 1972; Machado *et al.*, 1985; Wolfsdorf and Nolan, 1974; Leitzmann *et al.*, 1977; Rich, Neumann and Stiehm, 1977);
- thymic size in children with acute malnutrition (Nassar *et al.*, 2007; Naeye, 1965; Watts, 1969; Smythe *et al.*, 1971; Schonland, 1972; Aref *et al.*, 1982; Jambon *et al.*, 1988; Parent *et al.*, 1994; Chevalier *et al.*, 1994, 1998; Collinson *et al.*, 2003; Garly *et al.*, 2008; Moore, *et al.*, 2009; Chevalier, 1997).

Similarly, there are mixed results in studies of delayed-type hypersensitivity, although most communications report some impairment (Smythe *et al.*, 1971; Bhaskaram and Reddy, 1974, 1982a; McMurray *et al.*, 1981; Greenwood *et al.*, 1986; McMurray, Watson and Reyes, 1981; Seth *et al.*, 1981; Satyanarayana *et al.*, 1980; Heyworth, 1977; Smith *et al.*, 1977; Abbassy *et al.*, 1974; Harland, 1965; Puri *et al.*, 1980; Sakamoto and Nishioka, 1992; Kielman, 1977; Edelman, 1973; Geefhuysen *et al.*, 1971; Castillo-Duran *et al.*, 1987; Fakhir *et al.*, 1989; Schlesinger and Stekel, 1974; Ziegler and Ziegler, 1975). However, vaccine responsiveness appears unaffected by malnutrition (Savy *et al.*, 2009). In summary, SAM appears to increase the likelihood that a child will experience infections and that such infections will be more severe than in a child without SAM. However, the magnitude of the increased risk is only modest, as these infections occur in regions of the world with high incidences of infections, severe infections, and infection-related mortality in children without SAM.

The expert committee considered a panel of pathogens that cause illnesses of diverse severity in the context of childhood infections and the likelihood of their being transmitted by LMFs. Table 2 summarizes that analysis.

TABLE 2. Pathogenic micro-organisms considered in the hazard identification

Micro-organism	Reason for inclusion[1]	Syndrome	Seriousness of disease (h/m/l)[2]	Can manufacturing defects make ready-to-use foods (RUFs) a credible source of foodborne infections with the stated pathogen?[3]	Comments
Non-typhoidal *Salmonella*	1, 2	Gastroenteritis, sepsis, urinary tract infection (UTI)	High	Yes, because these agents have been found in product, they have been identified as causes of outbreaks related to low-moisture foods, the infectious dose is low, and the pathogen resists desiccation.	Non-typhoidal salmonellosis has been described in the settings of interest. While the documented distribution of serovars of *Salmonella* in human populations and RUFs are different, some serovars have been identified in both people and product. For example, the most common serotypes found in humans in the United States of America are Sandiego, Schwarzengrund, Panama, Heidelberg, Oranienburg, Poona, Enteriditis, Saintpaul, 1,4,[5],12:i:–¸ Agona, Infantis, Newport, and Javiana (Crump *et al.*, 2011). These differ from those found in product (Zanzibar, Mikawasima, Give, Koketime, Weltevreden) (P. McClure, personal communication). However, *Salmonella* Weltevreden (3) and *Salmonella* Mikawasima (4) have been recovered from humans in outbreaks
S. pneumoniae		Pneumonia, meningitis, sepsis	High	No. 2	This bile-soluble organism is an important pathogen in the population of concern, and not foodborne, but facilitates comparison of the seriousness of both foodborne and non-foodborne pathogens.
Klebsiella pneumoniae (and probably also *oxytoca*)	2	Pneumonia, sepsis, UTI, possibly gastroenteritis	High	No. 2, 5	No clear foodborne source, and very common in stools, food and environment. Most cases are associated with healthcare settings.
Citrobacter freundii	2	Sepsis, UTI	High	No. 2, 5	No clear foodborne source, and very common in stools, food and environment. Most cases are associated with healthcare settings.
Enterobacter spp. (not *Cronobacter*)	2	Sepsis, UTI	High	No. 2, 5	No clear foodborne source, and very common in stools, food and environment. Most cases are associated with healthcare settings.
Cronobacter spp.	1	Sepsis, meningitis	High	No. 1, 4	Most infancy cases are associated with healthcare settings.

Micro-organism	Reason for inclusion[1]	Syndrome	Seriousness of disease (h/m/l)[2]	Can manufacturing defects make ready-to-use foods (RUFs) a credible source of foodborne infections with the stated pathogen?[3]	Comments
Enterobacteriaceae (EB)	1	Not in strict sense	N/A	N/A	Indicates maintenance of hygienic practices and protection of product from contact with water.
Enterococcus spp.	2	Sepsis, UTI	High	No. 2	Indicator of faecal contamination
Listeria monocytogenes	1, 2	Sepsis, febrile gastroenteritis	High	No. 4	
Shigella	2	Yes	Moderate	No. 5	
Campylobacter	4	Diarrhoea	Low or moderate	Not further discussed	Pathogenicity is difficult to establish in settings of interest
Diarrheagenic *E. coli* (ETEC, EAggEC, EPEC, possibly EIEC, but not EHEC)	2	Diarrhoea	Moderate	No. 5	Pathogenic members are exceptionally difficult to define.
Bacillus cereus	4	Gastroenteritis	Moderate-high	No. 3, 4, 6.	*Bacillus* might require a different screening strategy
Clostridium *botulinum*	4	Flaccid paralysis	High	No. 3, 4, 6.	Not believed to be a problem in this age group
S. typhi and *S. paratyphi* B	2	Sepsis	High	No. 5	Not further considered
Toxigenic *Staphylococcus aureus*	1	Vomiting, diarrhoea	Moderate	Not further discussed	Pathogenicity is difficult to establish in settings of interest
Toxigenic *Clostridium perfringens*	1	Vomiting, diarrhoea	Moderate	No. 3, 4, 6	
Noroviruses	3	Vomiting, diarrhoea	Mild, moderate	No. 6	
Hepatitis A	3	Hepatitis	Mild, moderate	No. 6	

[1] 1 = legacy pathogen from 2012 report; 2 = serious pathogen based on continuing reports from paediatric centres in developing countries; 3 = common enteric viral pathogens; 4 = common bacterial pathogen that may be present in RUFs.

[2] High = potentially life-threatening; moderate = rarely life-threatening but might require visit to a care facility; low or mild = usually does not require a visit to a care facility.

[3] Reasons for not considering RUF manufacturing a likely cause for public health problems with this pathogen: 1 = pathogen does not affect children in age group of interest; 2 = not a foodborne pathogen; 3 = microbial physiology is not conducive to causing disease when ingested immediately from unopened product (i.e. will not sporulate or germinate in product); 4 = high doses needed to cause disease, usually requiring growth of the agent in the food; 5 = measures to control non-typhoidal *Salmonella* will control this agent; 6 = considered to be best controlled either before manufacturing at level of supplier or during preparation

3.2 HAZARD CHARACTERIZATION

Considering the preceding discussion, it was concluded that, on the basis of its ecology and documented ability to contaminate, survive in, and cause outbreaks of illness associated with LMFs similar to RUFs, *Salmonella* is the pathogen of most concern in RUFs. Accordingly, it was determined that management of the safety of RUFs for MAM and SAM consumers should focus on control of *Salmonella* in RUFs. It was further agreed that control of *Salmonella* would also be expected to reduce to an acceptable level the potential risk of illness from other foodborne pathogens, with the exception of spore-forming pathogens, that could commonly contaminate RUFs.

Salmonella cannot grow in LMFs owing to the low water activity, although the ability of *Salmonella* to persist in dry foods for long periods is well documented (see Section 3.3). Therefore, if salmonellae contaminate LMF products such as RUFs, they are likely to persist for months or even years, although gradual die-off will be seen over time. Higher storage temperatures result in a more rapid die-off. As such, the risk may be reduced during storage, and management of food safety risk does not need to "factor in" the potential for *Salmonella* to grow in the product before consumption unless the product is mixed with liquids that increase its water activity to $A_w = 0.94$ or higher, or produce a two-phase, water-in-oil emulsion.

To assess the risk from *Salmonella* in RUFs, and to develop appropriate food safety management guidance relevant to RUF processors and agencies responsible for administration of RUFs to children with MAM and SAM, it is necessary to develop an understanding of the relationship between the dose (numbers) of *Salmonella* potentially ingested in RUFs and the likelihood of onset and the severity of illness resulting from such potential exposures via RUFs.

Historically, based on data from volunteer human feeding studies involving healthy young adult males, it was concluded that typical doses required to cause illness were in the tens of thousands to tens of millions of cells. However, those studies were conducted on small numbers of subjects of the lowest susceptibility who were exposed under artificial conditions. As such, their responses are unlikely to be representative of the response of the population of interest for lipid-based RUFs. Moreover, outbreaks of naturally occurring salmonellosis associated with LMFs (Greenwood and Hooper, 1983; Craven *et al.*, 1975; D'Aoust *et al.*, 1975) and other food types (Vought and Tatini, 1998; Hennessy *et al.*, 1996; D'Aoust, 1985) have challenged the notion that foodborne salmonellosis requires ingestion of a very large dose, and numerous outbreaks with high attack rates have been attributed to foods contaminated at relatively low doses (e.g. only hundreds of cells or fewer per gram) (FAO and WHO, 2002; Teunis *et al.*, 2010; Boring, Martin and Elliot,

1971; Fontaine *et al.*, 1980; Fazil, 1996; Fontaine *et al.*, 1978; Ministry of Health and Welfare, Japan, 1999; Kasuga *et al.*, 2004; Matsui *et al.*, 2004; George, 1976; Lipson, 1976; Blaser and Newman, 1982). However, outbreak data are by their nature biased towards the responses of people who are most susceptible (Teunis *et al.*, 2010).

More recent research and expert opinion on foodborne infectious processes consider that even a single cell of a pathogen such as *Salmonella* has the potential to cause human infection (FAO and WHO, 2003), but that the probability generally is very low. Mathematical models to describe the probability of infection and illness related to the dose ingested have been developed. The "exponential" and "beta-Poisson" models both encompass the notion that the probability of infection is related to the dose ingested, that each cell has the ability to cause infection, and that the probability is not influenced by the total number of cells ingested. The beta-Poisson model adds the further consideration that some cells may be more, and some less, able than others to survive through the stomach and upper intestinal tract to be able to produce an infection, i.e. the beta-Poisson model assumes that there is a distribution of probabilities of survival, while the exponential model does not explicitly consider this possibility but considers only the average survival. However, in practice, both consider the role of biodiversity when subjected to consideration of the uncertainty associated with any measure of dose-response relations. One underlying assumption used in these dose-response models is that the severity of the disease manifestations is not associated with the dose ingested. However, Glynn and Bradley (1992) concluded that, while this assumption appeared valid for *Salmonella* typhi / typhoid fever, an association was observed between the severity of non-typhoidal *Salmonella* gastroenteritis outbreaks and ingested dose, possibly reflecting differences in pathogenesis of localized intestinal tract infections and systemic invasive infections. However, the data available to the expert committee do not allow differentiation of effects and, in general, the data suggest that exposure from RUFs will usually be very low doses.

Mathematical models relating the probability of non-typhoidal *Salmonella* gastroenteritis to the dose ingested in food have been developed and presented in the peer-reviewed literature by FAO and WHO (2002) and Teunis *et al.* (2010). Both are based on extensive data collated from outbreaks of salmonellosis in which it was possible to generate estimates of the doses ingested and proportion of consumers who developed symptoms of uncomplicated enteric salmonellosis. Figure 3 shows an example of the expected relationship between dose ingested and probability of gastrointestinal salmonellosis, based on the FAO/WHO (2002) model and variations. However, neither of these models differentiates the dose-response relationship according to food vehicle, and the food substrate may affect the dose-response relationship, for example, if the food provides protection to the cells during passage through the stomach and upper intestine, or if the conditions in the food, such as low water activity, induce enhanced resistance mechanisms in Salmonella cells in those foods.

While a continuous relationship exists between the dose of a pathogen ingested and the probability of illness, a convenient way of summarizing and comparing pathogen virulence is the concept of the ID_{50}, i.e. that dose (number of cells ingested) of a pathogen that would be expected to lead to an adverse clinical outcome in 50 percent of people who ingested that dose.

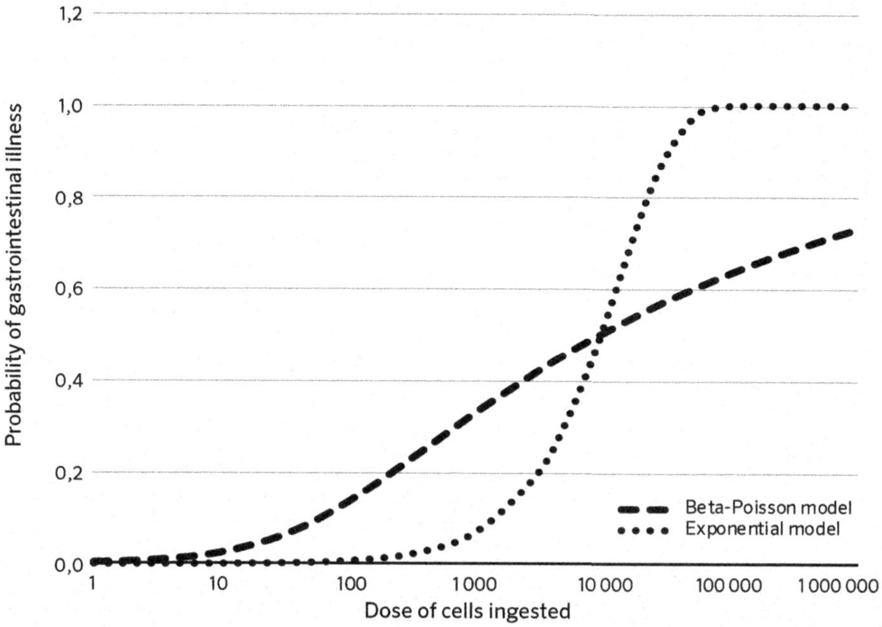

FIGURE 3. Examples of relationships between dose and probability of gastrointestinal non-typhoidal *Salmonella* infection

Note: The beta-Poisson model was fitted to available outbreak data (see FAO and WHO, 2002), while the exponential model was developed to have the same ID50 as the beta-Poisson model (see Annex 2). The plot illustrates that the choice of model can have a significant effect on predicted risk from low doses of *Salmonella*.

In Figure 3 the original FAO/WHO (2002) beta-Poisson model is shown as well as an exponential model that has the same ID50 as the FAO/WHO (2002) model. It is apparent that the analogous exponential model produces very different estimates of probability of illness for doses both higher and lower than the ID_{50}. Figure 4 shows the differences between the models at doses of from 1 to 100 cells – more likely to be relevant to the aims of the expert meeting. It is also noteworthy that while the exponential model assumes a constant, and simple, proportionality between dose ingested and probability of symptomatic illness, the beta-Poisson model predicts a more complex relationship between dose and probability of illness. It is apparent from Figure 4 that there are large differences in the two models at the low doses that are likely to be the most relevant to potential exposures from RUFs. Moreover, some of the curvature apparent in the model is derived because the "dose" data are plotted on a logarithmic scale, while the probability of illness scale is linear. When both dose and response are presented on a linear scale, the differences in the two models are more apparent, as shown in Figure 5.

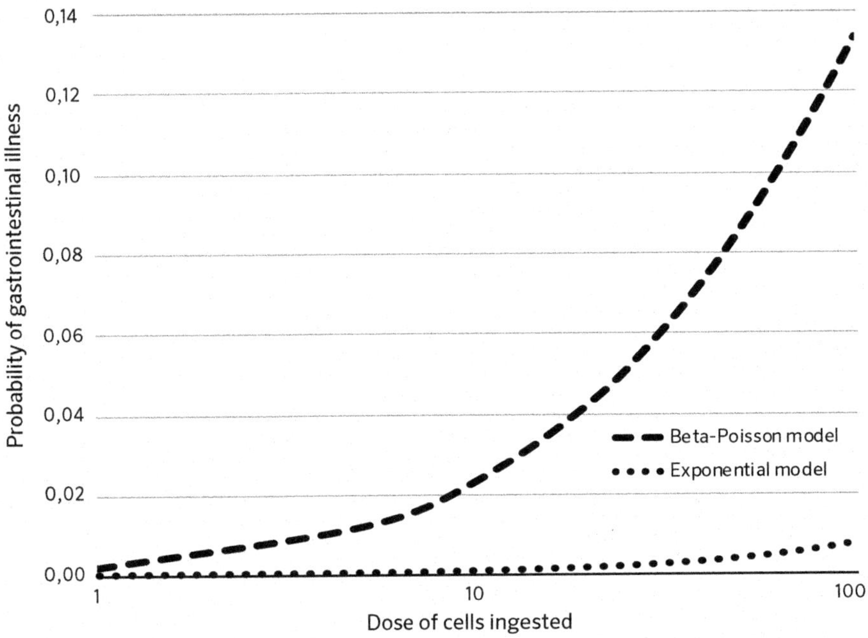

FIGURE 4. Examples of the predicted relationships between dose and probability of gastrointestinal non-typhoidal Salmonella infection from different models

Note: The dose scale is logarithmic, while the response scale is linear.

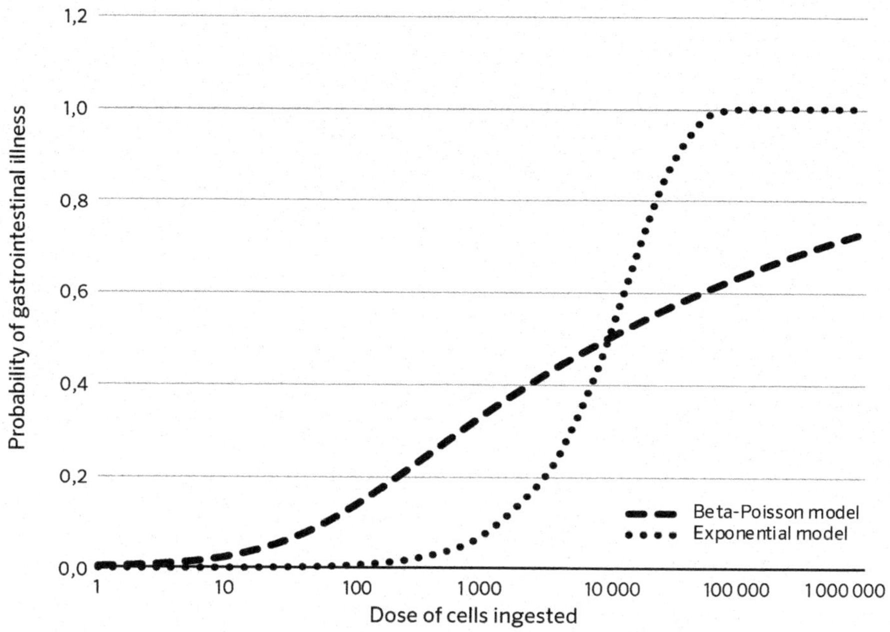

FIGURE 5. Examples of the predicted relationships between dose and probability of gastrointestinal non-typhoidal Salmonella infection from different models with both modelled responses shown on a linear scale

To place these differences between the two models into context, the data from the 23 outbreaks on which the FAO/WHO (2002) dose-response model are based, as well as the model itself, are presented in Figure 6, together with the analogous exponential dose-response model derived from the ID_{50} of the FAO/WHO (2002) model (see Annex 2).

Based on the various published models and analyses of additional data (see Annex 2) the estimated ID50 for *Salmonella* ranges from 36 cells to 1.4 million cells. These widely differing estimates are, in part, based on the choice of model as well as the databases used. For the peanut-butter-related outbreak (Cavallero *et al.*, 2011) and the potato-crisps outbreak (Lehmacher, Bockemuhl and Aleksic, 1995), only the exponential model can be used because there is only one estimate of dose and one estimate of the probability of illness. As illustrated above and in Annex 2 and 3, the choice of model, model assumptions, and dataset may lead to widely different estimates of the risk from *Salmonella* in foods, including RUFs, and, correspondingly, could lead to very different proposed strategies for risk management. Accordingly, the expert committee also attempted to develop dose-response relationships based on outbreaks related to LMFs most similar to RUFs, namely a peanut-butter-related outbreak in the United States of America affecting

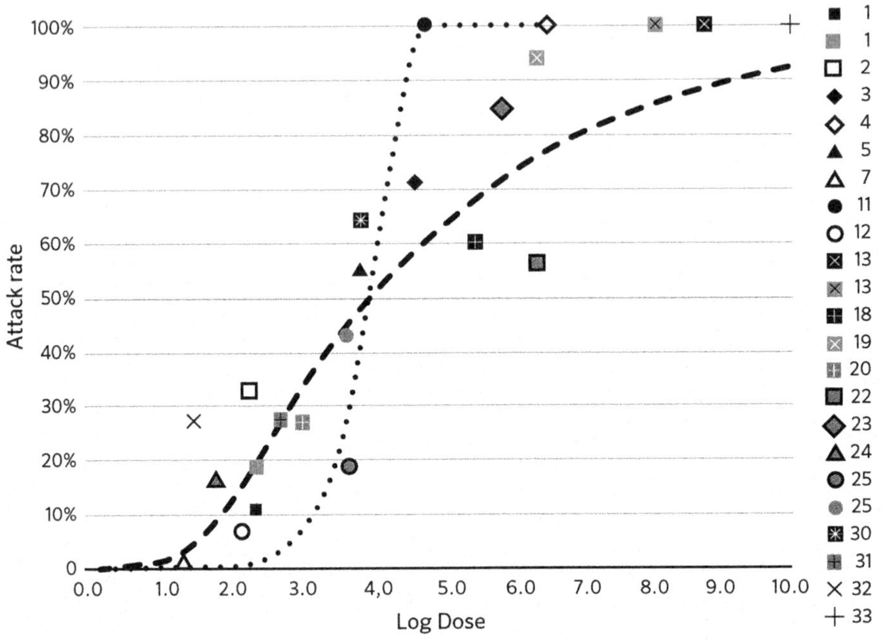

FIGURE 6. FAO and WHO (2002) "dose-vs-probability of gastrointestinal non-typhoidal salmonellosis" model

Note: FAO/WHO (2002) 'dose-vs-probability of gastrointestinal non-typhoidal salmonellosis' model and data from 23 outbreaks on which it is based (dashed line). Also shown is an analogous exponential model (dotted line) derived from the ID_{50} of the FAO/WHO (2002) model.

more than 700 people (Cavallero *et al.*, 2011), and an outbreak in Germany linked to Salmonella-contaminated paprika on potato crisps (Lehmacher, Bochemuhl and Aleksic, 1995).

The FAO/WHO (2002) model and analysis of the potato-crisps outbreak data (Lehmacher, Bockemuhl and Aleksic, 1995) lead to ID50 estimates in the range of 5 000–10 000 cells. The FAO/WHO (2002) dose-response model implies an ID50 of 9 600 cells and is based on the work of an expert group's analysis of 23 data (attack rates) from a diverse range of outbreaks, while the potato-crisp-related outbreak provides only a single attack rate related to one outbreak. It is not possible to derive a beta-Poisson model from a single observation, but an exponential model can be derived from one observation, and an ID50 estimated from it. Annex 2 present an analysis of the latter outbreak to generate ID50 estimates, including the assumptions made. The model of Teunis *et al.* (2010) is also based on the work of a diverse group of experts in modelling, risk assessment, epidemiology and public health, and an even larger set of outbreak data than the FAO/WHO (2002) model, and has also been presented in the peer-reviewed literature. However, the inferred ID50 is 36 cells, which does not accord with conventional experience, and leads to unexpectedly high estimates of numbers of cases observed in some outbreaks, including the potato-crisps outbreak mentioned above (Lehmacher, Bockemuhl and Aleksic, 1995). A re-analysis of the data presented in Teunis *et al.* (2010) was undertaken (see Annex 3) that considered the effect of assumptions used in the model-fitting process as well as minor transcription errors in the data presented in Table 1 of that report. The data in that report were fitted to a beta-Poisson model, i.e. the same type of model as used for the FAO and WHO (2002) model. The beta-Poisson model fitted to the corrected Teunis *et al.* (2010) dataset is virtually identical in the low dose range to the FAO/WHO (2002) model, as shown in Figure 7. Under one assumption about the variance in the data, both models fitted to a beta-Poisson model generate ID50 values of about 10 000 cells. Importantly, both show similar predictions in the very low dose regions expected to be relevant to RUFs, based on the existing test results database.

A further model, developed by Bollaerts *et al.* (2008) using the same data as used by FAO/WHO (2002), was not considered because the results cannot be easily generalized for use in risk assessment studies owing to the complexity and specificity of the models and attendant data needs.

Conversely, estimates based on the anecdotal data available for the peanut-butter-related outbreak in the United States of America in 2008–09 (Cavallero *et al.*, 2011) suggest an ID50 estimate of about 800 000 cells, even though peanut butter is an LMF that might be expected to protect *Salmonella* from inactivation during passage through the stomach and small intestine. This estimate is derived from a single outbreak involving a single strain, which may have been of unusually low virulence. Moreover, the data could only be fitted to an exponential model, as discussed above. Given these large differences in model estimates of ID50s and the consequent effects on risk estimates, a decision was made to use the FAO/WHO (2002) dose-response model because of the quantity of data that it is based on, because it has been subject to peer review (with a history of use since 2002), and because of its consistency with ID50 estimates developed from the paprika-seasoned potato crisp-related outbreak and the re-analysed Teunis *et al.* (2010) dataset. However, it must be noted that the decision to adopt the model for the risk assessment leading to proposed sampling plans for lipid-based RUFs was not able to be based on incontrovertible evidence that the FAO/WHO (2002) model is the best representation of the average probability of infection of humans exposed to different levels of an unspecified strain of *Salmonella*. Rather, it was selected because it was agreed that, all things considered, the FAO/WHO (2002) is currently the most defensible dose-response model for non-typhoidal *Salmonella* gastroenteritis.

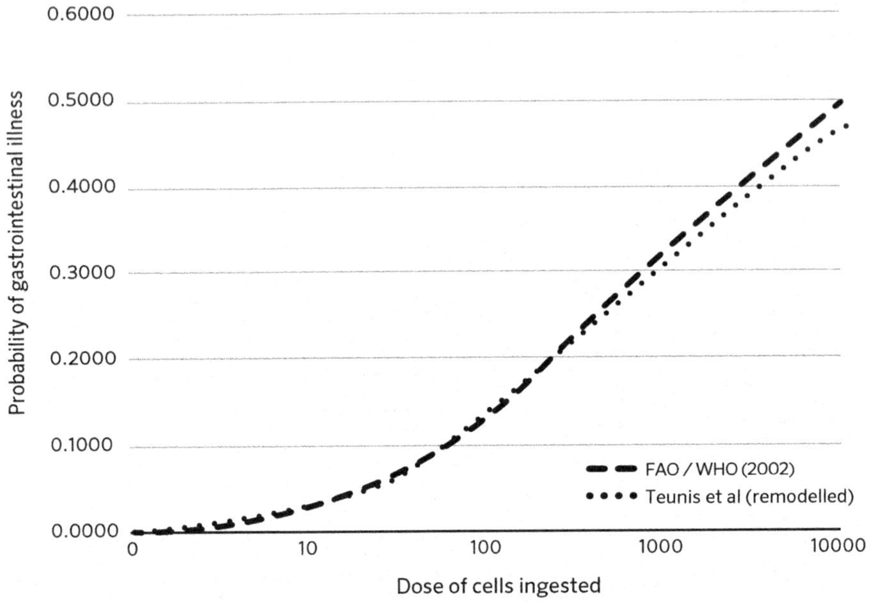

FIGURE 7. FAO/WHO (2002) "dose-vs-probability of gastrointestinal non-typhoidal salmonellosis" model compared with a beta-Poisson model fitted to the expanded salmonellosis database (after correction for transcription errors) presented in Teunis *et al.* (2010)

However, the FAO/WHO (2002) model does not specifically consider children, who may have increased susceptibility owing to SAM. It is noteworthy that analysis of the outbreak data used to generate the FAO/WHO (2002) model could not demonstrate that "susceptible" populations, including children less than five years old, are more likely to acquire salmonellosis from a given dose, although that report did add the caveat that it is possible that more susceptible people have more severe cases of salmonellosis, as discussed above. Similarly, Teunis *et al.* (2010), while specifically analysing for differences in response due to expected pre-disposing susceptibilities and developing separate models for responses among susceptible and "non-susceptible", observed that the "non-susceptible and susceptible models developed here are very similar."

From the available published data (see Section 3.1), the expert committee inferred that acutely malnourished children between the ages of 6 months and 59 months may be as much as 2–5-fold (on average 3.5-fold) more susceptible than are children of the same age without malnutrition (Berkowitz, 1984; Norton *et al.*, 2004; Bronzan *et al.*, 2007; Bachou *et al.*, 2006; Berkley *et al.*, 2005). This range of relative susceptibility may be within the margin of safety commonly achieved by ready-to-eat LMFs produced by major food manufacturers for the general population. Therefore, the expert committee considered that standards for similar LMFs produced for the general public serve as good points of reference for raw-ingredient and finished-product standards for lipid-based RUFs.

Nonetheless, the expert committee also attempted to deduce relevant MC using a quantitative "risk assessment" approach. This employed the FAO/WHO (2002) model but modified the model, or its predictions, to reflect this increased susceptibility, i.e. the modified model assumed that SAM children are 3.5 times more likely to develop a gastrointestinal salmonellosis from a given dose, noting that this approach is only valid in the low dose range.

3.3 EXPOSURE ASSESSMENT

Foods with Aw < 0.60, including lipid-based RUFs, do not support the growth of micro-organisms. Bacteria capable of causing foodborne illness cannot grow in foods at Aw < 0.85. However, micro-organisms can survive for many months, even years, in low-Aw foods and dry environments in which foods and food ingredients may be stored (Beuchat *et al.*, 2013; Podolak *et al.*, 2010; Burnett *et al.*, 2000; Keller *et al.*, 2013; Santillana Farakos, Frank and Schaffner, 2013). Proaña-Peralta *et al.* (2011) reported that Salmonella survived on raw peanut kernels for at least 26 weeks under their experimental conditions. Burnett *et al.* (2000) observed that Salmonella survived in peanut butter (Aw = 0.20–0.33) for at least 24 weeks under their experimental conditions.

Among the population of micro-organisms that may be initially present in low-A_w foods, only a small proportion exhibits this ability to survive for long periods. Fluctuation in temperature and exposure to stresses such as acid pH and naturally occurring antimicrobials in foods with Aw less than that required for growth may enhance the rate of inactivation. The rate of die-off of *Salmonella* and other foodborne pathogens is reduced as the Aw of foods and storage temperature are decreased (Burnett *et al.*, 2000). For example, Beuchat and Mann (2010) stored pecan nutmeats with an Aw of 0.51–0.63 at 4 different temperatures between –20 °C and +37 °C. In pecan halves and pieces contaminated with 2.56 log CFU/g of a five-strain cocktail of *Salmonella* serotypes, the nutmeats stored at –20 °C and +4 °C experienced very small reductions in *Salmonella* levels after 52 weeks of storage, whereas those stored at +37 °C decreased significantly after 2 weeks and decreased further between 2 weeks and 24 weeks. With storage at either +21 °C or +37 °C, *Salmonella* were detectable only by enrichment after 52 weeks of storage. Therefore, if salmonellae contaminate LMF products such as RUFs, they are likely to persist for months or even years, particularly if they are stored at low temperatures to prevent rancidity during storage (Burnett *et al.*, 2000). However, if low-Aw foods such as RUFs are mixed with high-Aw foods, *Salmonella* and other foodborne pathogens that are present may grow. High numbers of pathogens may develop within a few hours, depending on storage temperature, pH, and nutrient availability. This can result in an increased risk of illness to the consumer.

As *Salmonella* does not grow in lipid-based RUFs, a reasonable estimate of frequency and extent of exposure of young children to *Salmonella* from consuming contaminated product can be made by determining the frequency and extent of contamination at the time of manufacture. This would be considered a worst-case estimate, as there is likely to be some reduction in *Salmonella* levels as a result of product storage prior to consumption.

Currently, limited *Salmonella* data exist for RUFs, with various manufacturers having widely different rates of testing, apparently using a variety of methods and sampling plans. Based on the data provided to the expert committee (more than 4 000 test results for products from 21 suppliers), the rate of positive samples ranged from a high of 1 in 5 samples to a low of 0 in 393 samples. The expert committee was not able to estimate the levels of contamination in the positive samples because the analyses were limited to presence/absence testing. However, a low frequency of detection in samples from the same process implies a low mean log concentration of the target micro-organism. Based on the data provided, the percentage of servings contaminated with *Salmonella* ranges from approximately 0.2 percent to 20.0 percent among the various manufacturers, with an average rate of about < 0.5 percent, calculated from the 23 positive results from all survey data available to the expert committee from the agencies, based on their own analyses and those of the manufacturers, involving 4 448 samples in total (personal communications from WFP, UNICEF, MSF and participants of the Paris RUF suppliers meeting, October 2014). When the survey data from each agency were considered separately, each produced an average *Salmonella*-positive rate of between 0.4 percent and 0.9 percent.

In the absence of data on the relative proportion of the total production supplied by each manufacturer, it was not possible to calculate the overall exposure rate, because some manufacturers may be consistently more likely to produce *Salmonella*-contaminated RUFs. Similarly, the available data did not allow the expert committee to distinguish the impact of intervention technologies (e.g. thermal pasteurization) as the details of the individual suppliers' processes were not provided.

The expert committee was also provided with data on the levels of EB assessed in more than 10 000 samples (personal communications from WFP, UNICEF, MSF and participants of the Paris RUF suppliers meeting, October 2014). The food industry uses EB extensively as an indicator micro-organism for the level of hygienic practices used to control microbiological contamination in dry products manufacturing. The three-class plan currently implemented by the purchasers indicated that levels between > 10 and < 100 CFU/g would be considered marginally acceptable, and levels > 100 CFU/g would be considered unacceptable. Using those criteria, approximately 1.3 percent of samples were manufactured under marginally hygienic conditions, and approximately 0.3 percent of the samples produced under unhygienic conditions. No data were presented at the meeting that allowed the expert committee to determine the degree of association between unhygienic manufacturing conditions and incidence of *Salmonella*-positive servings.

The low level and frequency of contamination that currently exists in RUFs (based on the survey data) should be noted in the context of the method and environment of feeding. As the product is provided to young children either on the caregiver's finger or squeezed directly from the sachet to the child's mouth, the finger and external surface of the sachet could be contaminated, and it is possible that these external sources could be more important for exposure to *Salmonella* than is the current level of contamination of the product itself. It is not unreasonable to consider the efficacy of the manufacturing-level risk mitigations in relation to mitigations appropriate to other sources of exposure. However, no data assessing these avenues of exposure were available to the expert committee; therefore, it was not feasible to disaggregate the possible exposures of children being fed lipid-based RUFs to estimate the likely role of current levels of *Salmonella* in the product in causing illness. In addition, epidemiological follow-up of infections occurring during nutritional management of SAM and MAM is generally not attempted.

3.4 RISK CHARACTERIZATION

There is a high degree of uncertainty concerning both the hazard characterization (i.e. dose-response relationship) and the exposure assessment described above. Thus, any quantitative risk characterization based on those assessments will also have a high degree of uncertainty. Nonetheless, some inferences are possible from those analyses, including the probability, based on the low frequency of *Salmonella*-positive samples, that contamination levels in RUFs are low, e.g. typically only one or a few cells per serving and, therefore, that those doses are in the "linear" portion of the dose-response curve (see Figure 5). In this region, for a tenfold reduction in the dose (or concentration) of *Salmonella* in a serving, a tenfold reduction in the probability of illness is expected. Thus, any mitigation that achieves a 1-log reduction in the average level of *Salmonella* will reduce the risk of illness tenfold, whether gastroenteritis or bacteraemia. That said, these inferences would not hold true if the contamination were not randomly distributed within the food or if some contaminated servings of RUFs contained very high levels of *Salmonella*. However, this is unlikely in a homogeneous product such as RUFs, in which processing would be expected to distribute any contaminants more uniformly throughout the product and in which any contaminating *Salmonella* cells are unable to grow. As an example, the observation that approximately five 25-g samples in every 1 000 (0.5 percent prevalence) contain one or more *Salmonella* cells suggests that approximately 1 in every 200 sachets (of about 100 g each) will contain one or more *Salmonella* cells at the point of manufacture. Assuming that the concentration of *Salmonella* is log-normally distributed with a standard deviation of $0.5\ log_{10}$CFU (because the product is well mixed, the standard deviation of the counts in the product is assumed to be 0.5 [van Schothorst *et al.*, 2009]), then the expectation would be for approximately 1 in 3×10^6 servings of 100 g to contain 10 or more cells, and approximately 1 in 10^{13} servings to contain 1 000 or more cells of *Salmonella.*

While substantial microbiological data were provided to the expert committee on a presence/absence basis, levels of *Salmonella* as well as uncertainty about the sensitivity of the methods employed in generating those data make it difficult to estimate the probability of illness with a high degree of confidence. Nonetheless, the data can be used to consider the range of risk likely to be encountered. For example, if it is assumed that *Salmonella* is present in a sachet at a level of 1–10 CFU per serving, and that the frequency of contaminated servings ranged from < 0.2 percent to 20 percent (see above), then the approximate risk of salmonellosis can be calculated by substituting 1 or 10 into the dose-response equation and then considering the cumulative probability of illness to a SAM child from multiple exposures to potentially contaminated servings in a specified period. Assuming that the child is consuming 2 servings a day for a period of 31 days (a total of 62 servings), and that the child is 3.5 times more likely to develop an infection from a low dose of *Salmonella*, the estimated risk of gastrointestinal salmonellosis, for different scenarios, is presented in Table 3. As is evident from the table, the probability of salmonellosis is expected to decrease dramatically as the extent and frequency of contamination is reduced.

TABLE 3. Examples of the predicted risk of gastrointestinal salmonellosis for SAM children receiving a full course of RUFs (62 servings) based on different levels and frequencies of RUF contamination

Colony-forming units (CFU) / serving	Percentage contaminated servings	Probability of salmonellosis after 62 servings
1	< 0.2	< 0.0011
	20.0	0.10
10	< 0.2	≤ 0.010
	20.0	≤ 0.64

Note: Calculations are based on the FAO/WHO (2002) dose-response model, adjusted by 3.5 for SAM children susceptibility.

Within the ranges specified above, substituting other values for extent of contamination per serving and frequency of contamination can be used to provide an estimate of probability of salmonellosis.

As a simple example, let the assumption be that the RUF serving is 100 g and the goal is that ≤ 2 percent of sachets, or ≤ 0.5 percent of sachets, contain one cell of *Salmonella* (N.B. the scenario is approximately the current situation). Using the same dose-response model as above, the estimated probabilities of gastrointestinal salmonellosis after consuming 62 servings are ≤ 0.010 and ≤ 0.0028, respectively. If a tolerable level of risk can be agreed upon, this can be used to establish a presence/absence sampling plan that could ensure this level of risk is not exceeded, based on available statistical knowledge and tools. First estimates are possible using the binomial distribution, but tend to very slightly overestimate the number of samples required (Ross *et al.*, 2011). More sophisticated and accurate treatments are possible using online tools developed by FAO/WHO (www.fstools.org/sampling/) and the International Commission on Microbiological Specifications for Foods (ICMSF) (van Schothorst *et al.*, 2009).

Using the first example, these requirements indicate that to be 95 percent confident that a lot of product does not have ≥ 1 CFU/serving in 2 percent of servings, and thus be a non-conforming batch to be detected and rejected, would require the analysis of 149 sachets, all of which would need to be negative for *Salmonella*. The relationship between the numbers of samples analysed for this example and the probability that despite the testing the lot would be accepted is depicted in Table 4.

TABLE 4. Relationship between the number of 100 g servings analysed and the probability of accepting a contaminated lot

Number of sachets analysed	Estimated likelihood that the lot would be *accepted* if it had ≥ 1 *Salmonella*/serving in 2% of the servings (%)	Estimated likelihood that the lot would be *accepted* if it had ≥ 1 *Salmonella*/serving in 0.5% of the servings (%)
1	98.0	99.5
2	96.0	99.0
5	90.4	97.5
20	66.8	90.5
50	36.4	77.8
100	13.3	60.6
149	5.0	47.4

To be sure that the frequency of contamination did not exceed 0.5 percent would require testing of 598 sachets and for all to be shown to be free of *Salmonella*. At these levels, the expected probabilities of gastrointestinal salmonellosis among SAM infants would be 1 in 90 children if 2.0 percent of sachets were contaminated, or 1 in 360 children receiving a course of RUFs if 0.5 percent of sachets were contaminated.

This simplified example clearly indicates that, as the required target level of risk is reduced, the use of microbiological end-product testing as a control step (i.e. test and release microbiological testing) becomes increasing impractical. That is, sampling and testing of food products are effective tools to verify compliance with preventive and sanitation programmes, process control and sanitary conditions, HACCP-based systems, and microbiological criteria, but sampling and testing food products are inefficient and ineffective means to guarantee food safety. Achieving low risk levels with manufactured products typically involves the inclusion of intervention steps, such as a pasteurizing or sterilizing technology, which substantially reduce or eliminate pathogen loads in the product. In such instances, confirmation of effectiveness is by other means (e.g. examination of time/temperature profiles), with microbiological testing being focused on process verification and control of re-contamination of the food.

4

Managing the risk of salmonellosis from lipid-based RUFs fed to children 6–59 months of age with MAM and SAM

4.1 RISK-BASED FOOD SAFETY MANAGEMENT

The ability to consistently produce a product that manages microbiological risks to the degree discussed above requires four areas of active control: (i) maintenance of GHPs; (ii) raw-ingredient sourcing controls; (iii) inclusion of appropriate intervention technologies; and (iv) prevention of re-contamination.

4.1.1 Good hygienic practices

Good hygienic practices (GHPs) provide the basic factors that need to be controlled for the production of foods. These include factors such as the design and layout of the manufacturing facility, training of employees, and general sanitation procedures. The basic code of hygienic practice (CAC, 1969), and the more recent Codex Code of Hygienic Practice for Low-moisture Foods (CAC, 2015), are available from Codex Alimentarius and are useful documents. Similarly, the Grocery Manufacturers Association's Guidelines for Controlling *Salmonella* in Dry Foods (GMA, 2009) has information that should provide RUF manufacturers with useful approaches to addressing their concerns. Additional sources of information that are likely to be helpful to RUF manufacturers are the GHPs and GMPs for products, such as peanut butter, with similar attributes and processing technologies. As dry products, RUFs face significant challenges in cleaning and sanitization. The manufacturers need to be fully cognizant that uncontrolled wet cleaning of manufacturing facilities can increase the likelihood of *Salmonella* in the facility and in the products they produce.

4.1.2 Raw ingredients

As currently manufactured, RUFs undergo differing degrees of processing based on the technologies being employed. If the technologies employed do not include a lethal intervention step, selection of raw-ingredient suppliers becomes a critical step in the production of safe product. Ongoing active assessment of the capabilities of potential suppliers to continuously provide raw ingredients with adequately controlled levels of *Salmonella* contamination should be part of any supplier agreement. Manufacturers of RUFs should consider requiring certificates of analysis for key raw ingredients. Moreover, periodic verification of raw-ingredient suppliers' ability to meet the purchase specifications should be performed by the RUF manufacturer or a third-party laboratory. This control can be enhanced if the agency or other purchasers of the final product require access to the results of such raw-ingredient testing by the RUF manufacturer.

4.1.3 Intervention technologies

The risk of salmonellosis can be actively reduced by the inclusion of appropriate treatments to reduce the levels of *Salmonella* (and other pathogens) in the product. The most commonly used and cost-effective technology is thermal processing, although there are other possibilities. This type of dry product represents a challenge owing to the increased thermal resistance of micro-organisms as water activity is reduced. However, considering that each tenfold reduction in *Salmonella* levels will produce a tenfold decrease in risk, an inactivation treatment of 4–5 log cycles will produce a 10 000–100 000-fold decrease in risk of salmonellosis. This, in combination with careful selection of raw materials with minimal levels of contamination, should ensure production of a low-risk product. It is worth noting that as a major component of most RUF formulations is peanuts, ensuring proper roasting coupled with preventing re-contamination should provide low-risk raw materials, which will help ensure that even a moderate intervention step will be highly effective.

4.1.4 Re-contamination

As with any processed product, the effectiveness of intervention steps is only as great as the safeguards put in place to ensure that the product does not become re-contaminated. Typically, this is achieved through a combination of GHPs and specific barriers put in place to minimize potential cross-contamination. This includes proper zoning to control access of pathogens to post-treatment product, and is enhanced through use of sealed systems after thermal treatment that minimize potential exposures until the product can be packaged in the sealed sachets. There is a substantial body of knowledge about the protocols and technologies available to minimize re-contamination of products such as RUFs that can be accessed to develop appropriate procedural and physical barriers to re-contamination.

4.2 THE ROLE OF MICROBIOLOGICAL TESTING IN FOOD SAFETY MANAGEMENT

Microbiological testing of foods or food ingredients is an integral part of most food safety systems, but the specific approach to testing is highly dependent on the type of food safety management system that a company or an industry is implementing. Assuming that an industry is applying Codex Alimentarius Commission guidelines for the production of lipid-based RUFs, companies should be employing a GHP/HACCP-based risk management system for ensuring microbiological safety. Typically, the approach to microbiological testing will be either lot-based testing (LBT) of end products (or key ingredients) as part of a "test and release" programme for the ingredients or finished product (FAO and WHO, 2016b), or process control verification (PCV) testing as part of a company's HACCP verification programme. The latter is typically part of a "cross-lot" testing programme that focuses on trend analysis. While the specific microbiological method used in both LBT and PCV may be the same, the means of sampling and the interpretation/response to the results are distinctly different. Buchanan and Schaffner (2015) have reviewed the difference between these two types of testing programmes in the context of microbiological testing for verification of preventive control systems, and key considerations related to the two types of testing programmes are summarized below.

Traditional end-product testing was originally designed to examine food lots (typically at ports of entry) for which there was little information available on how the food had been manufactured. Thus, the purpose of the testing in this instance was to "prove" that a lot of food was safe. However, in modern food safety systems, there is a wealth of information available concerning the history and handling of foods. Despite this increased knowledge, a substantial number of manufacturers continue to employ "test and release programmes." It is important to note that when microbiological testing is performed in this manner, the testing becomes a de facto critical control point. The limiting factor in employing microbiological testing in this manner is that the number of samples needed to have confidence that one has actually identified a lot contaminated at an unacceptable level becomes very large when the percentage of servings that are contaminated falls below 2 percent. For example, to be 95 percent confident that < 2 percent of RUF servings are free of salmonellae requires that approximately 150 servings be tested and found negative for every batch. However, given the scale of production, if even 20 percent of units or RUFs were contaminated, many infants could become ill. Acceptable levels of protection are more likely to be 1 in 1 000 units (0.1 percent), or fewer, contaminated with *Salmonella*. At this level of prevalence, tens of thousands of samples needs to be tested and shown to be free of detectable levels of Salmonella, to ensure the overall safety of the lot.

Thus, as has been emphasized in this report, as the level of contamination (both frequency and concentration) decreases, the value of end-product testing to assure product safety is greatly diminished. In practice, end-product testing is now used primarily by the food industry and its regulators as an indicator of overall process integrity rather than individual lot integrity because, at the level of contamination control currently achieved by (and required of) food manufacturers, end-product sampling does not reliably distinguish lots that are unacceptably contaminated from compliant, safe lots.

Figure 8 helps illustrate that contaminated lots will be confirmed by almost any stringency of end-product sampling for manufacturers that have no control of their process and almost consistently produce contaminated lots. However, these manufacturers should be ruled out by observations and analyses conducted during preliminary on-site inspection. At the other extreme, for manufacturers that consistently operate at acceptable levels of process control, increasing the stringency of end-product sampling has virtually no impact on product safety. It is only in the middle of the contamination range, where manufacturers are not able to consistently maintain process control and occasionally produce lots that exceed safety specifications, that increasing the stringency of end-product sampling may enhance the likelihood of demonstrating loss of process integrity and indicate the potential for increased risk of consumer illness. Motivating RUF manufacturers in this last category to move up to consistent process control should be the overarching priority of all interactions between the purchasing agencies and the manufacturers of RUFs. The significance/relevance of "Case 14", "Case 11", 'status quo", and the appropriate level of protection (ALOP) referred to in Figure 8 are explained below.

In a GHP/HACCP-based food safety management system, one relies on preventive controls and intervention technologies to ensure that microbiological hazards are controlled to a desired level of protection. In such systems, a number of key processing metrics are "monitored" to ensure that the system is functioning within specifications. Typically, such measurements are physical (e.g. temperature) or chemical (e.g. pH, and water activity) in nature and can be done in real time. In addition, HACCP programmes require the use of appropriate verification

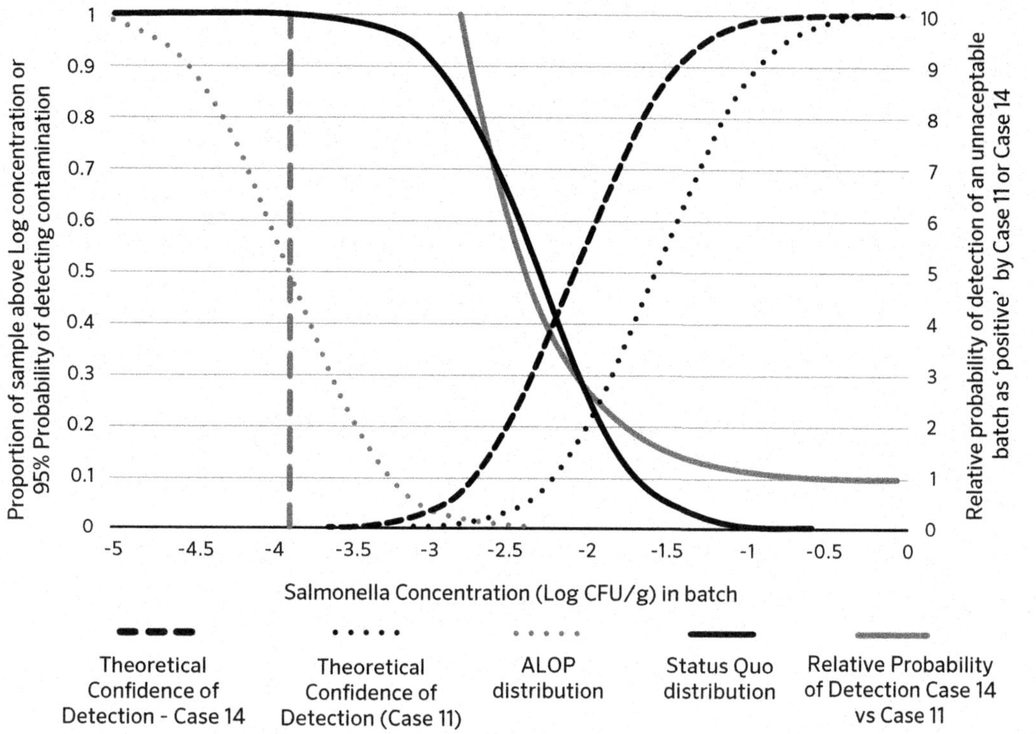

FIGURE 8. The relative sensitivity of different sampling plans to detect contamination of RUF meals by different levels of *Salmonella* and their relationship to realistic contamination levels. (The 'Status quo distribution' line represents the current expected level of contamination of RUF meals with Salmonella, based on survey data. It shows that the average contamination level (50th percentile) is ~1 cell per 200 g. At that level of contamination the 95% probability of detecting the contamination using a Case 11 sample plan (10 samples, all negative for Salmonella) is shown by the 'Case 11' line, and is ~5%. Increasing the sample plan stringency to Case 14 (30 samples, all negative for *Salmonella*), increasing the probability of detecting an 'above average' batch to ~30%. More importantly, however, at the desired level of (just) 'acceptable' contamination (ALOP distribution lines) either sampling plan has a probability of detection of an unacceptable batch of much less than 1%, i.e., the sampling plans are relatively ineffective. The green line shows the relative sensitivity of a Case 11 or Case 14 sampling plan for the existing distribution of contamination. However, if we determine that the ALOP should be an average of ~1 per 8000 g (ALOP distribution line) neither a Case 11 nor Case 14 can offer assurance of detection of an unacceptably contaminated batch of food.)

protocols. These are typically not real-time in nature (i.e. they require six or more hours) and are only performed periodically. The purpose of the verification testing is not to prove that any specific lot is safe, as that is done by the company's activities to monitor the process. Instead, the purpose of verification testing is to ensure that the food safety system has not changed and is under control. As a simple example, one can consider manufacture of a food product that relies on a thermal treatment (e.g. cooking) for a specified time and temperature to reduce the potential presence of foodborne pathogens to an acceptable degree. The safety of production lots of the food would be determined by monitoring the time and temperature of the thermal processing step. A key event occurs when the monitoring values are all within specifications but the verification testing indicates that the process is out of control. There are several potential interpretations of such findings, such as: (i) the incoming raw materials had significantly elevated levels of contamination that exceeded the capability of the thermal process; (ii) there has been an increase in the thermal resistance of the target micro-organism; (iii) a new source of post-thermal treatment re-contamination has arisen; (iv) the thermal treatment is not functioning despite the monitoring data (e.g. switch from turbulent to laminar flow); and (v) the process is in control and the positive finding was the result of a low-probability detection of the low-level residual prevalence of the target micro-organism. Buchanan and Schaffner (2015) identified a number of parameters related to the attributes of a fit-for-purpose PCV programme that have to be considered in terms of specific applications. These parameters include:

- What micro-organisms should be tested for in a PCV programme?
- Who should do the testing?
- What should be the frequency of testing?
- Where along the production process should the testing be performed?
- What corrective actions should be taken if PCV testing exceeds established levels?
- What is the role of environmental testing in PCV testing programmes?
- What actions should be taken if a performance criterion for a PCV testing programme is repeatedly exceeded?

One of the parameters emphasized for PCV testing of ready-to-eat products is the desirability of testing for an appropriate indicator micro-organism (Buchanan and Schaffner, 2015). From the standpoint of a regulatory agency responsible for overseeing the production of safe food products in relation to infectious micro-organisms such as *Salmonella*, if a pathogen is detected, the product should not be released into commerce and should be recalled if already released. Thus, for ready-to-eat products such as lipid-based RUFs, it is more desirable to test for appropriate indicator micro-organisms that are associated with increased risk of conditions associated with poor hygienic practices or faecal contamination that, in turn, would imply an increased risk of microbial hazards. The advantage of an indicator micro-organism is that it provides a means of detecting and correcting process deviations before a safety-based criterion is exceeded. The consultation reviewed several potential indicator micro-organisms, with assays for EB or non-pathogenic E. coli exhibiting a number of the characteristics that would make them viable indicator micro-organisms.

Based on the profile of manufacturers of lipid-based RUFs provided to the expert committee during the expert consultation, the industry can apparently be divided into:

- facilities that are manufacturing product under a GHP-only system based on sanitary controls;
- facilities that have applied the principles of risk management based on GHPs plus HACCP, including preventive controls and intervention steps to reduce the risk of microbiological contamination.

Thus, food safety management based on the current status of the industry would argue for two different types of microbiological testing specifically suited for each current type of process control. For the GHP-only facilities, this would entail implementation of microbiological testing programmes based on rigorous monitoring of the ingredients and production environment, plus lot-based "test and release" of individual production lots. While testing end products for pathogens is demonstrably insensitive for identifying contaminated lots, without the ability to develop a positive verification history of successful application of validated intervention technologies, more reliable statistical trend analyses as an indication of food safety are not possible. Conversely, for those facilities that have effectively implemented a GHP/HACCP risk management system with effective monitoring and verification programmes, the use of PCV testing is a scientifically justifiable and economically advantageous alternative. The approach of using different microbiological criteria for companies employing GHP-only versus GHP/HACCP food management systems has been used by national governments (e.g. differential requirements of the Food Safety and Inspection Service of the United States Department of Agriculture for *Listeria monocytogenes* testing). While the nutritional need of the subpopulation that is being served by this niche product is well understood, the principles and recommendations of the Codex Alimentarius Commission and many national governments regarding the desirability and feasibility of safe production of all foods must be considered. Accordingly, the expert committee suggested that the purchasers and users of lipid-based RUFs provide assistance and encouragement to aid the current GHP-only manufacturers to acquire as quickly as possible the knowledge, skills and resources to become GHP/HACCP facilities.

It is critical that the manufacturers of lipid-based RUFs understand the appropriate role of microbiological testing in food safety risk management so that they can participate in the establishment of adequate and appropriate GHP-only monitoring and testing, and GHP/HACCP-based verification testing programmes in the short term, with the ultimate goal of moving all RUF manufacturers to GHP/HACCP-based programmes. The purchasing agencies, FAO and WHO, can facilitate this transition by providing training and other assistance to lipid-based RUF manufacturers, particularly those in developing countries.

4.2.1 Setting a microbiological criterion

Microbiological criteria have been used in the food industry for many years and have contributed to improving food hygiene and safety in general, even when based on empirical observation of what can be achieved with existing measures without any explicit link to specific levels of public health protection. Advances in microbiological risk assessment, and the use of the risk management framework are increasingly allowing a more quantifiable estimation of the public health risk and a determination of the effect of interventions.

Microbiological criteria should be established in the context of risk management options and in accordance with the Principles and Guidelines for the Establishment and Application of Microbiological Criteria Related to Foods (CAC, 1997). As noted in the previous section, the microbiological safety of foods is managed by the effective implementation of control measures that have been validated, where appropriate, throughout the food chain to minimize contamination and improve food safety. Establishing MC can be appropriate for verifying that food safety control systems are implemented correctly and performing as required (CAC, 1997).

A number of approaches have been applied to developing MC. These range from developing MC based on empirical knowledge related to GHPs, to using scientific knowledge of food safety control systems such as through HACCP, and to establishing a dose-response curve and conducting a risk assessment. The choice of approach should be aligned with the risk management objectives and decisions relating to food safety and suitability (CAC, 1997). This latter point highlights the importance of the role of risk managers in the establishment of MC. Therefore, the Expert Group considered that, rather than simply providing a specific microbiological criterion and sampling plan, it was more appropriate to outline different approaches to establishing MCs that might be appropriate under different conditions, and how they could be applied in this particular context using the available information.

Further information on the statistical aspects of microbiological criteria related to foods can be found in the publication *Statistical Aspects of Microbiological Criteria Related to Foods* (FAO and WHO, 2016b).

4.2.2 Example approaches to setting a microbiological criterion for ready-to-use foods

Microbiological criteria can be established to serve a number of purposes. As indicated above, these include evaluating a specific lot of ingredients or finished food to determine its acceptance or rejection, and to date this has been the most common application of MC for RUFs. This use of criteria has value, particularly if an ingredient supplier or manufacturer of RUFs does not have an established safety history. However, it indicates only that any likely contamination is below the specified level, but does not guarantee absence of contamination. Another purpose of MC is to provide information to food business operators on microbiological levels that should be achieved when applying best practices. In the case of RUFs, this is a way for the purchasing agencies to communicate their requirements to the suppliers. However, with a move to a preventive approach, a more practical application of MC is for verifying the performance of a food safety control system or its elements along the food chain, e.g. PRPs and/or HACCP systems. This allows the MC to be used in a different way and to consider data accumulated over time using different methods of trend analysis, such as control charts and moving windows. Such an approach can be beneficial in that it allows a record of safe production to be established, anomalies and occasional contamination events to be identified, and a better overall understanding to be obtained of the performance of the process, and, therefore, of the safety of the product. This information can serve to better assure and improve the performance of the process.

Linking an MC to risk and the level of protection it provides to consumers requires some articulation of an ALOP. In the absence of a stated ALOP, it is not possible to use the hazard characterization and exposure assessment information to deduce a relevant MC for RUF products administered to children with SAM. However, if an ALOP is established, no practical level of end-product sampling can come close to assuring absence of pathogens at that level; hence, alternative safety assurance approaches must be employed.

The Expert Group attempted a number of approaches, three of which are presented below to illustrate the process and expected sampling plan that would be required. These approaches are provided to assist risk managers in making a decision, but not to suggest to them what the ALOP is, or the appropriate sampling plan to achieve it.

Approach 1. Reference to existing criteria

In the absence of a scientifically based ALOP, it may be possible to develop a sampling plan based on an analogous product that takes into account any differences in the product or the consumers being exposed. A sampling plan of n = 10 × 25 g samples, c = 0 for particular categories of LMF (peanut butter, chocolate, cocoa powder and confectionary products) has been proposed by the ICMSF (2011) and termed a "Case 11" sampling plan. Given the characteristics of some of these products, they can be considered analogous to lipid-based RUFs and thus form an appropriate reference point for establishing an MC for lipid-based RUFs.

Given the data reviewed, the Expert Group estimated that SAM children are approximately 3.5 times more susceptible to *Salmonella* infections than are other children in the community who are not malnourished (see Section 3.2). Therefore, the recommended sampling plan for RUFs should provide confidence that the product being consumed by SAM children is 3.5 times less likely to contain any *Salmonella*, or that the average *Salmonella* level must be 3.5 times lower than the tolerable level for normal-weight, healthy children. Relating these requirements to existing analogous criteria suggests that approximately 3.5 times more product should be tested and found to be free of *Salmonella*. This requirement is met, approximately, by an n = 30 ×25 g, c = 0 sampling scheme, sometimes described as an ICMSF "Case 14" sampling plan.

With this approach, purchasing agencies may hope that the presence of an MC with a rigorous sampling plan will encourage manufacturers to maintain a level of process control adequate to result in infrequent positive test results. Over time, this should improve the level of safety of RUFs and decrease the likelihood of RUF-associated foodborne disease. However, the safety approach of applying an MC for an analogous product is used without knowledge of how much it may reduce the risk of illness among RUF consumers.

Approach 2. Deriving a sampling plan from a putative ALOP

Another basis for establishing MC that has been used in other regulatory setting processes requires imputing an ALOP by determining a socially acceptable incremental risk of illness that would be added by the product to the pre-existing endemic risk of that illness from all other sources. However, doing so, requires an estimate of the "endemic" risk, in this case the background rates of uncomplicated gastrointestinal salmonellosis or *Salmonella* bacteraemia unrelated to exposure to RUFs. Global estimates of gastrointestinal illness are difficult to calculate for many reasons, especially because many countries, particularly developing countries, have insufficient surveillance data (Majowicz *et al.*, 2010). This appears to be changing, at least in some regions (Page *et al.*, 2013; Langendorf *et al.*, 2015), but will require massive increases in resources for laboratory and surveillance infrastructure to establish global data for food safety decision-making.

It is known that the risk of gastrointestinal illness varies by age and region (Majowicz *et al.*, 2010; Scallan *et al.*, 2005). From telephone surveys of more than 34 000 people in four developed countries, Scallan *et al.* (2005) found that about 2.1 percent (weighted mean) of people experience symptoms of gastroenteritis in any four-week period, when disease was defined as diarrhoea (> 3 loose stools in 24 hours) persisting for more than 3 days. Using this relatively strict definition of gastrointestinal disease, an annual risk of gastroenteritis of 27 percent, i.e. approximately one in four people per year, can be derived. Moreover, the data indicate that children under 5 years old are about 1.56 times (weighted mean) more likely than the general population to experience symptoms of gastroenteritis, i.e. they have a 42 percent probability of gastrointestinal illness per year. In developing countries where children with SAM live, the probability of gastrointestinal infections is somewhat higher. Kosek, Bern and Guerrant (2003) and WHO (2013b) report that, in developing countries, children under the age of 5 years have, on average, three episodes of diarrhoea every year.

There are various estimates of the specific contribution of salmonellosis to this disease burden. Scallan *et al.* (2005) estimated that 3 percent of gastrointestinal infections in developed nations were due to *Salmonella*, while the data of Page *et al.* (2013) suggest that among children admitted to hospitals in Niger with complicated severe acute malnutrition, about 10 percent yielded Salmonella on culture from their stools, whether diarrhoea was evident or not. Similarly, Langendorf *et al.* (2015) found that in children with moderate to severe diarrhoea in Niger, about 10 percent yielded Salmonella from stool samples whether the diarrhoea was watery or bloody. If mixed infections were excluded, the prevalence of *Salmonella* in stools was 4.8 percent (watery diarrhoea) or 6.7 percent (bloody diarrhoea).

From the above, it is possible to estimate that the endemic risk of infection to which children in developing countries might be exposed would result in three cases of gastroenteritis per year, and that about 10 percent of the risk will be from *Salmonella* infections, i.e. a probability of uncomplicated enteric salmonellosis of 0.3 cases per year. Using the SAM-modified FAO/WHO (2002) dose-response model, assuming that contaminated sachets contain only one cell of *Salmonella*, and assuming consumption of 62 sachets of RUFs, up to 66 percent of servings could contain a single cell of *Salmonella* and not exceed that "endemic" level of risk of enteric salmonellosis. That would involve a doubling of risk of salmonellosis for consumers of lipid-based RUFs (i.e. endemic risk plus the additional risk from a course of RUFs) (see also Section 3.4). However, if an incremental risk of 10 percent of salmonellosis were considered socially acceptable, the frequency of *Salmonella*-contaminated sachets should be less than one sachet out of about 18, or approximately < 1 *Salmonella* per 1.7 kg of RUFs. To demonstrate with 95 percent confidence that this criterion was met would require testing about 50 sachets. The best evidence available to the Expert Group indicates that salmonellae are currently present at low concentrations in about 0.5 percent of samples tested. Using the modified FAO/WHO (2002) model to account for the increased susceptibility of SAM children, the present average risk of uncomplicated gastrointestinal salmonellosis for a child with SAM who receives a course of 62 servings of RUFs is estimated to be 1 in about 350 SAM (about 3 per 1 000, 0.3 percent) children, i.e. approximately a 10 percent increase in risk over the endemic level.

As stated previously in this report, the aetiology of uncomplicated gastroenteritis is difficult to determine in the settings where lipid-based RUFs are used. Therefore, the Expert Group attempted to look instead at the incremental risk of *Salmonella* bacteraemia and sepsis, conditions that can be aetiologically confirmed. Data exist that suggest that approximately 1 percent of enteric non-typhoidal salmonellosis will progress to invasive disease (Hohmann, 2015). Accordingly, perhaps 1 in 35 000 (about 0.03 per 1 000) children with SAM who are administered a full course of lipid-based RUFs could develop *Salmonella* bacteraemia or sepsis from exposure to contaminated RUFs. While the resource-intensive epidemiological studies necessary to document such a low risk have not been reported, the experience of paediatricians caring for children with SAM to whom the expert committee had access (both expert committee members and resource persons) suggests that the risk of invasive salmonellosis decreases and does not increase during nutritional management of acute malnutrition with lipid-based RUFs.

It has been noted that non-typhoidal salmonellosis is becoming a more common cause of invasive disease in Africa (Graham, 2010; Feasey *et al.*, 2012), and that this seems to be associated with serovars of *Salmonella* that are more prevalent in Africa. The serovars of *Salmonella* that may contaminate lipid-based RUFs should reflect those common to the source of RUF ingredients and the RUF production environment. Therefore, if the proportion of RUFs manufactured in Africa increases, both the endemic risk of *Salmonella* bacteraemia and sepsis and the incremental risk associated with administration of RUFs could change. Re-evaluation of these risk estimates and appropriate levels of protection and sampling plans may be required if production significantly increases in the region in which the invasive strains are more prevalent.

Approach 3. Process verification sampling for RUF product using the moving window technique

The above approaches are based on the testing of product on a lot-by-lot basis. An alternative approach that can be highly effective, particularly in manufacturing facilities that apply proactive prevention or intervention steps to reduce or minimize *Salmonella* levels, is the use of PCV testing (ICMSF, 2002; Buchanan and Schaffner, 2015). As discussed above, this method is an HACCP-based risk management approach of monitoring real-time physical or chemical measurements of the interventions used to control *Salmonella*, with microbiological testing focused on verifying that the controls and the overall food safety system are continuously operating as intended. For example, process verification sampling for the RUF product with the same sensitivity as the traditional ICMSF end-product sampling could employ a "moving window" sampling plan that involves using an eight-sample moving window. It is important to keep in mind that control of the process is being continuously verified in this approach through physical and chemical tests and assays for indicator micro-organisms, and that the assays for pathogens in the moving window serve as an overview of the safety of the entire process and reassurance that the assumptions underlying process design remain valid. In this approach, the eight samples (a sample is considered a 25 g analytical unit) are taken over a specified number of days or shifts. For example, it could be extended to 1 sample per day with an 8-day window, 4 samples per day with a 2-day window or, if doing two production shifts per day, it could be 2 samples per shift per day with a 2-day window. The specific combination selected is dependent on the needs of the manufacturers. However, eight samples taken over shorter periods of time allows more rapid detection of a loss of process control, and will result in less product being discarded when deviations occur.

In this example, it is assumed that c = 0 and that 4 samples per day are analysed in conjunction with a 2-day window. Thus, if the samples for the first and second day are all negative, the process is considered in control. The window then moves by one day and the results for days 2 and 3 are considered. If no *Salmonella*-positive sample is detected on day 3, the process continues to be considered "in control." However, let it be presumed that on day 4 that one of the four samples is positive. There would then be a 2-day window (days 3 and 4) in which c = 0 has been exceeded and the production process is deemed out of control.

Part of the immediate response when this occurs is to put the product produced during that specific window on hold, perform a "root cause analysis" and make the appropriate corrections. The product produced during the deviation would be discarded. Presuming that the root cause analysis has successfully identified the sources of the deviation and appropriate corrective actions have been carried out, production could restart, but the manufacturer must re-establish the "under control" moving window. Product produced as the manufacturer is re-establishing the "under control" 2-day window should be held until such time that the 8-sample window has no positive *Salmonella* finding. It is worth noting that the longer is the original window selected, the longer it will take to return to "in control status" after a process deviation. If the manufacturer is confident that it has identified and corrected the root cause, it may consider doing enhanced testing (e.g. quadruple the number of tests per day or shift) to provide assurance that the system has returned to its baseline level of performance. A manufacturer that has ongoing moving window failures of the verification testing should re-evaluate its HACCP plan, as this is indicative of an improper consideration of one or more risk factors, missing one or more critical control points, or a breakdown in the good hygienic and manufacturing practices needed in any food production setting. Similarly, continuing inability of a manufacturer to meet verification testing requirements should trigger an audit and review by the purchasing agencies or organizations.

This safety assurance approach, based on assurance of the integrity of a validated process, can be used in the presence of an ALOP established on the basis of a consumer-specific dose-response curve and complete risk assessment. However, it also is helpful in the absence of an ALOP if a validated process can be continuously verified because it is more sensitive to potential contamination than end-product sampling, and it identifies loss of control more quickly, which allows rapid termination of potentially unsafe production and identification of causes of deviation.

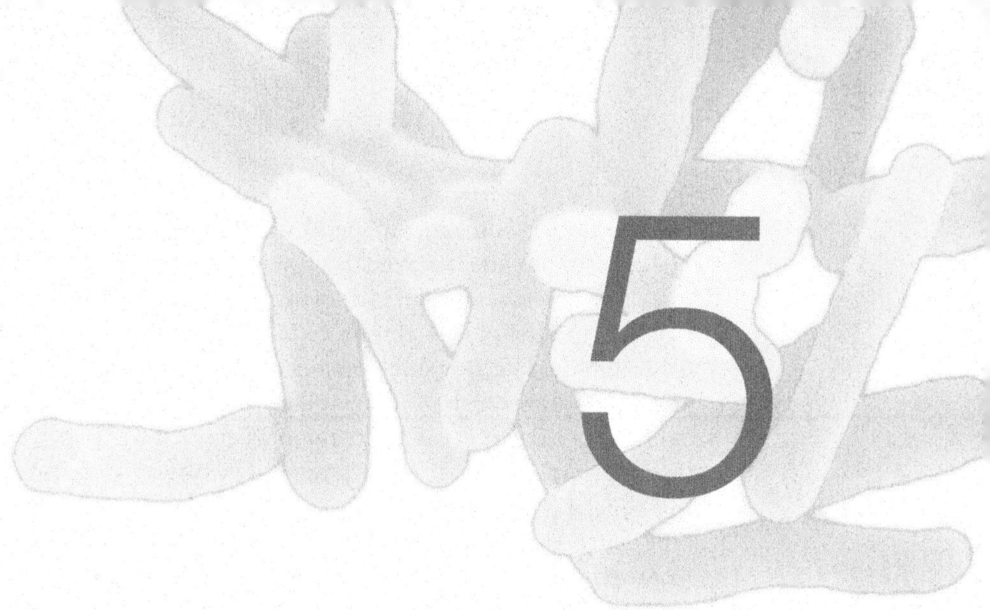

5

Conclusions

5.1 PATHOGEN(S) OF CONCERN

1. The expert committee began its deliberations by conducting a microbiological hazard identification for RUFs. This review included a large range of bacterial pathogens that are potentially present in RUFs, and other bacterial and viral pathogens that have been identified as causes of life-threatening infection in children within the target population for RUFs and could also be foodborne. As a result of this review, the expert committee strongly reaffirmed the conclusion of the 2012 expert consultation that *Salmonella* is the "highest priority infectious hazard and its control in lipid-based RUF the most important microbiological food safety programme goal" (FAO and WHO, 2016a). Moreover, after careful consideration, the expert committee considered that, with the exception of spore-forming pathogens, other bacterial pathogens would be adequately controlled by food safety measures adopted to reduce the risk from *Salmonella*.

5.2 SUSCEPTIBILITY OF CHILDREN WITH SAM RELATIVE TO CHILDREN OF THE SAME AGE WITHOUT MALNUTRITION

2. The expert committee agreed with the findings of the 2012 expert consultation that "malnutrition deranges all of the body systems of a child" and increases both the probability of infectious diseases and the risk of

serious adverse outcomes of infections. From the available published data the expert committee inferred that acutely malnourished children between the ages of 6 months and 59 months may be 2–5-fold more susceptible (average 3.5 fold), but almost certainly not more than fivefold more susceptible to infection from foodborne pathogens than are children of the same age without malnutrition. This range of relative susceptibility may be within the margin of safety commonly achieved by similar ready-to-eat, low-moisture, processed foods produced by major food manufacturers for the general population.

3. The target population for lipid-based RUFs is likely to be exposed to serious pathogens, including *Salmonella*, from multiple sources (e.g. other foods, water, animals and the surrounding environment). The expert committee concluded that the risk of foodborne illness posed by lipid-based RUFs produced under the conditions and to the standards recommended by the expert committee is likely to be very low in comparison with the risk of infections from other sources, given the available information, which suggests that, on average, less than 1 percent of RUF servings are contaminated with low levels of *Salmonella*. However, the expert committee also noted the paucity of substantial aetiological and epidemiological data on the population of interest that are available to make such judgments with confidence.

5.3 ASSESSING THE PROBABILITY OF FOODBORNE INFECTION FROM RUFS

4. Lipid-based RUFs will not support growth of pathogens. In fact, product characteristics are more likely to lead to die-off of vegetative pathogens, with the rate increasing with temperature of storage. However, even at warm ambient temperatures, inactivation by this "passive" process is slow, and a tenfold reduction in *Salmonella* concentration might take many months to occur.
5. The data from EB testing generated at the recommendation of the 2012 expert consultation suggest that 98–99 percent of RUF samples comply with the current EB criterion, with less than 1 percent above 100 CFU/g (M value). It is noted that the EB sampling plan recommended by the 2012 expert consultation is either consistent with, or more stringent than, existing sampling plans for similar products marketed globally by leading manufacturers to the "general" consumer population.
6. Data from *Salmonella* testing by the producers and agencies suggest that less than 1 percent of portions of RUFs contain *Salmonella* and that, when

present, the levels appear to be very low, i.e. between 1 and 10 viable cells per contaminated serving. Using the FAO/WHO (2002) dose-response model and assuming that the child is consuming 2 servings a day for a period of 31 days (a total of 62 servings), and that the child is 3.5 times more likely to develop an infection from a low dose of *Salmonella*, the estimated risk of gastrointestinal salmonellosis, for different scenarios was estimated. While serovar and host immune status influence the likelihood of progression from gastrointestinal infection to more severe forms of salmonellosis, less than 10 percent of gastrointestinal illnesses predicted by either dose-response model are likely to progress to bacteraemia and life-threatening illness.

7. Following implementation of the food safety recommendations in the 2012 report, substantial production improvements have been achieved overall, and collaborative relationships have been established between suppliers and purchasing agencies that should result in reduction in the likelihood of RUFs containing gastrointestinal pathogens. Some suppliers have implemented pathogen inactivation steps for some "higher-risk" raw materials (e.g. peanuts) used in RUF manufacture. As far as is known, no suppliers have implemented an in-line intervention that would be considered a final kill step.

5.4 POTENTIAL TO IMPLEMENT KILL STEPS TO FURTHER REDUCE MICROBIAL CONTAMINATION

8. Limited thermal inactivation data generated using a strain of *Enterococcus faecalis* and multiple strains of *Cronobacter* species in lipid-based RUFs indicate that as much as a 3-log reduction in enteric pathogens can be consistently achieved using temperatures between 75 °C and 130 °C. Decimal reduction times (D values) at 80 °C can be up to 1 hour, while at temperatures in the range of 120–130 °C, D values of about 6 seconds have been reported. These data are consistent with other studies reporting thermal inactivation of pathogens, including *Salmonella*, in other LMFs (e.g. with A_w = 0.4–0.5).
9. In addition to conventional thermal pasteurization, technologies that show promise for substantially reducing *Salmonella* in lipid-based RUFs without causing unacceptable loss of quality of the product, e.g. radio frequency treatment, are being evaluated for their efficacy in enhancing microbiological safety of LMFs.

5.5 MICROBIOLOGICAL CRITERIA APPROPRIATE TO LIPID-BASED RUFS AND HOW THEY SHOULD BE USED

10. Implementation of recommendations from the 2012 expert consultation for out-of-specification EB counts are judged to be no longer the most effective means of achieving continuous improvement in the microbiological safety of lipid-based RUFs. It is noted that EB counts are generally recommended for process assessment/trend analysis, and not as end-product safety criteria. The expert committee reiterates that the EB criteria are appropriately used as a hygiene indictor wherein elevated levels lead to investigation of the process by the manufacturer to identify and eliminate the cause of increased contamination. For analogous products, EB levels of < 100/g are typically achievable.

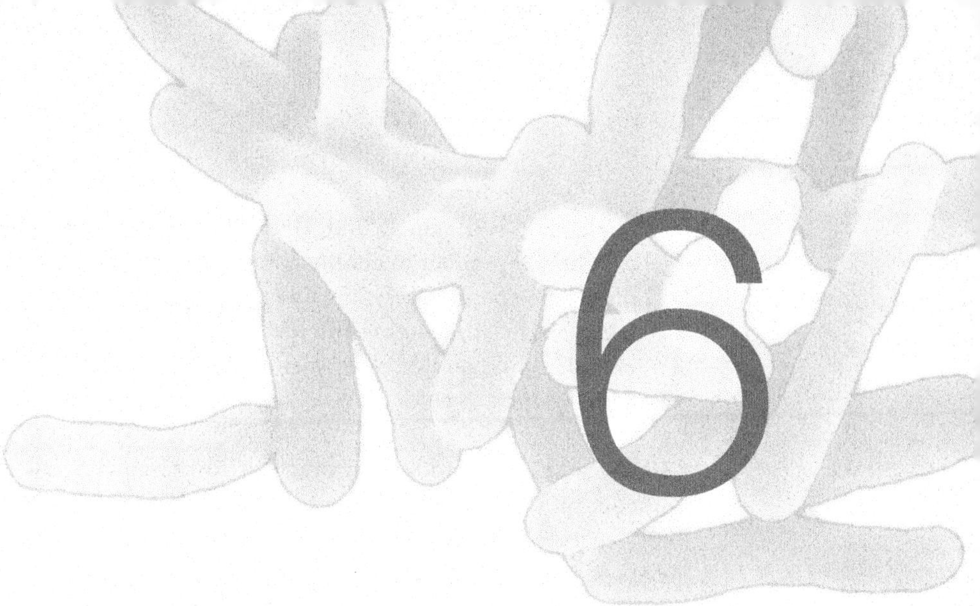

6

Recommendations

6.1 RECOMMENDATIONS FOR MANUFACTURERS

1. Manufacturers should adopt and document proven food safety management strategies, such as the HACCP approach, to increase and maintain the microbiological safety of RUFs. As noted, current data suggest that the main foodborne infectious hazard in LMFs, including lipid-based RUFs, is *Salmonella*. Action to prevent contamination with *Salmonella* should also control contamination with other relevant vegetative microbial hazards.

2. Most RUF manufacturing processes do not currently include a kill step for relevant microbial hazards in the final product. Accordingly, the food safety programme should ensure that ingredients are sourced from suppliers with adequate control measures for control of *Salmonella*, and that there are validated measures in place in the processing environment to control *Salmonella*. For example, manufacturers should:
   - procure raw ingredients only from suppliers that can assure the consistent microbiological safety of those ingredients, and, especially for processes that do not include a validated kill step, reject raw ingredients with elevated EB counts;
   - maintain the product and ingredients in a dry state, limit the use of water in the production environment, and ensure that any wet cleaning of equipment is accompanied by thorough drying before it is reassembled;

- implement PRP, GMP and GHP protocols, and ensure adequate blending of product to eliminate foci within the lot that have enough moisture to permit growth of *Salmonella;*
- take steps to eliminate vermin that could carry *Salmonella;*
- exclude food handlers with gastrointestinal infections from working with product.

3. Zoning and other production practices to prevent re-contamination of product should be strictly observed following application of a validated kill step, especially one that is documented to achieve ≥ 5 log reduction in levels of *Salmonella*.

4. The strategies and actions taken to ensure absence of *Salmonella* should be documented by each manufacturer, and all workers should be trained in those strategies.

5. The safety of the manufacturing process used in each facility should initially be validated by microbiological testing of final product, ingredients and the processing environment. Thereafter, the level of process control and product safety should be continuously evaluated and periodically verified to assess whether the food safety controls are functioning as intended. Continuous evaluation should be done by monitoring control points against pre-established criteria as part of a documented monitoring plan that includes adherence to the principles of GMPs, implemented through a safety monitoring system based on HACCP with appropriate PRPs and operational PRPs.

6. Manufacturers should establish written operational goals that ensure the safety of lipid-based RUFs for malnourished children, and specify corrective actions if there are marginal hygiene evaluation findings, including microbiological testing results for EB. These corrective actions to critical deviations include, but are not limited to, root cause investigations and adherence to corrective action plans. This documentation would be expected to include details of sampling programmes and methods to ensure the microbiological safety of ingredients and the production environment.

7. Manufacturers should continue to investigate and implement, as appropriate, changes in processes and new technologies that will consistently achieve reductions in *Salmonella* and other pathogens of interest necessary for full implementation of HACCP.

6.2 RECOMMENDATIONS FOR AGENCIES

1. Programmes that use lipid-based RUFs should maintain a focus on *Salmonella* as the highest-priority infectious hazard, and its control as the primary food safety programme goal.
2. Revisions to the MC / sampling plans recommended in the 2012 report may be considered based on data generated since 2012. Criteria for *Salmonella* in similar ready-to-eat LMFs with potential for contamination with *Salmonella* but that do not allow its growth (e.g. nut butter, and chocolate) involve an n = 10 (× 25 g samples), c = 0 sampling plan (ICMSF Case 11). This could be adopted for RUFs; but in doing so, it is important to be aware of the limitations of MC and the associated sampling plan. The difference in susceptibility of the intended consumer compared with the general population could be somewhat accounted for in the development of a more stringent plan (e.g. n = 30 [× 25 g samples], c = 0 sampling plan [ICMSF Case 14]).
3. End-product "hold and release" testing provides less assurance of product safety than does establishing and maintaining a safe process that includes prevention and intervention steps to control *Salmonella* through control of raw materials, process design and process steps that actively reduce *Salmonella* contamination of the product. Therefore, agencies should encourage and assist manufacturers currently using GHP/GMP-only processes with end-product test and release to upgrade to HACCP and PCV programmes. Workers should be trained in and demonstrate knowledge of the *Salmonella* control procedures, and manufacturers should monitor and document compliance with those procedures. The inclusion of intervention steps that actively reduce *Salmonella* contamination (e.g. pasteurization) should be a priority consideration, with monitoring and documentation of treatment parameters (e.g. time and temperature of a heat treatment), and inclusion of periodic microbiological sampling to verify the effectiveness of the control systems. This should include periodic verification testing of the product and the production environment. This can be done through periodic lot testing using an n =10 (× 25 g samples), c = 0 sampling plan, or a process control approach that provides an equivalent level of sensitivity (see Approach 3 in Section 4.2.2). Both monitoring and verification documentation should be reviewed on a routine basis by both the manufacturer and the purchasing agencies.
4. Testing the product and/or the processing environment is often a useful tool for the manufacturer to anticipate and thus prevent problems. Using an EB criterion (n = 10, c = 2, m = 10 CFU/g, M = 100 CFU/g) as a microbiological indicator can often help identify and correct process

deviations and hygiene lapses before there is *Salmonella* contamination of product. Deviation from the EB standard should not automatically lead to product rejection if subsequent rigorous *Salmonella* testing is negative and if review of the environmental monitoring programme and other aspects of the food safety system reveal no uncorrected deficiencies. Continuing deviations from the EB MC should lead to complete re-evaluation of the hygiene controls, including a re-evaluation and possible re-validation of the GMP/GHP and HACCP plans.

5. Continued training of suppliers and manufacturers is required in order to raise their awareness of the expectations of the agencies, the processing and product standards they need to meet to prevent RUF-associated infections of malnourished children, the ways in which they can effectively meet these requirements through process design and operation, and how they can demonstrate compliance. To achieve continuous improvement, such training may need to be followed by site-specific expert advice, leading to individualized changes in processes, procedures, documentation and facilities.
6. Education of manufacturers and their testing laboratories is needed regarding the implementation and conduct of tests required for process validation and monitoring, particularly in relation to appropriate methods of pooling of samples and the reporting/interpretation of results.
7. If lipid-based RUFs are mixed or added to other water-containing foods, such as porridge, microbial growth may become possible after re-hydration and further storage or holding. While the risk may be low under some conditions, users should be discouraged from using RUFs in this way, or be educated to consume them quickly if water or high-moisture food is added.
8. Agencies should determine whether it is possible or feasible to establish an infectious disease surveillance programme that can be followed in the field for children consuming lipid-based RUFs. Typical signs and symptoms of enteric infections and systemic spread of possibly foodborne disease following administration of lipid-based RUFs should be monitored and recorded, and promptly reported to the agencies for analysis of evidence of RUF-induced gastrointestinal illness or systemic infections. For those children identified as suffering from non-typhoidal salmonellosis, serotyping or genotyping of organisms causing infection should be undertaken and compared with serotypes isolated from production lots of lipid-based RUF products distributed within the programme area.

References

Abbassy, A.S., el-Din, M.K., Hassan, A.I., Aref, G.H., Hammad, S.A., el A. II., el-Din, A.A., Soliman, M.H. & Hussein, M. 1974. Studies of cell-mediated immunity and allergy in protein energy malnutrition. 1. Cell-mediated delayed-hypersensitivity. *Journal of Tropical Medicine and Hygiene,* 77(1): 13–17.

Altay, C., Bingol, A., Say, B. & Dogramaci, N. 1972. Nitroblue tetrazolium test in children with malnutrition. *Journal of Pediatrics,* 81(2): 392–393.

Annan, R., Webb, P. & Brown, R. 2014. *Management of moderate acute malnutrition (MAM): current knowledge and practice.* CMAM Forum Technical Brief. 39 p. (available at www.ennonline.net/attachments/2289/MAM-management-CMAM-Forum-Technical-Brief-Sept-2014.pdf).

Aref, G.H., Abdel-Aziz, A., Elaraby, II., Abdel-Moneim, M.A., Hebeishy, N.A. & Rahmy, A.I. 1982. A postmortem study of the thymolymphatic system in protein energy malnutrition. *Journal of Tropical Medicine and Hygiene,* 85(3): 109–114.

Bachou, H., Tylleskär, T., Kaddu-Mulindwa, D.H. & Tumwine, J.K. 2006. Bacteraemia among severely malnourished children infected and uninfected with the human immunodeficiency virus-1 in Kampala, Uganda. *BMC Infect Diseases,* 6: Article 160.

Beatty, D.W., Napier, B., Sinclair-Smith, C.C., McCabe, K. & Hughes, E.J. 1983. Secretory IgA synthesis in Kwashiorkor. *Journal of Clinical & Laboratory Immunology,* 12(1): 31–36.

Behrens, R.H., Lunn, P.G., Northrop, C.A., Hanlon, P.W. & Neale, G. 1987. Factors affecting the integrity of the intestinal mucosa of Gambian children. *American Journal of Clinical Nutrition,* 45(6): 1433–1441.

Berkley, J.A., Lowe, B.S., Mwangi, I., Williams, T., Bauni, E., Mwarumba, S., Ngetsa, C., Slack, M.P., Njenga, S., Hart, C.A., Maitland, K., English, M., Marsh, K. & Scott, J.A. 2005. Bacteremia among children admitted to a rural hospital in Kenya. *New England Journal of Medicine,* 352(1): 39–47.

Berkowitz, F.E. 1984. Bacteremia in hospitalized black South African children. A one-year study emphasizing nosocomial bacteremia and bacteremia in severely malnourished children. *American Journal of Diseases of Children,* 138(6): 551–556.

Beuchat, L.R. & Mann, D.A. 2010. Factors affecting infiltration and survival of *Salmonella on in-shell pecans and pecan nutmeats. Journal of Food Protection,* 73(7): 1257–1268.

Beuchat, L.R., Komitopoulou, E., Beckers, H., Betts, R.P., Bourdichon, F., Fanning, S., Joosten, H. M. & Ter Kuile, B.H. 2013. Low-water activity foods: Increased concern as vehicles of foodborne pathogens. *Journal of Food Protection,* 76(1): 150–172.

Bhaskaram, C. & Reddy, V. 1974. Cell mediated immunity in protein-calorie malnutrition. *Journal of Tropical Pediatrics and Environmental Child Health,* 20: 284–286.

Bhaskaram, P. 1980. Macrophage function in severe protein energy malnutrition. *Indian Journal of Medical Research,* 71: 247–250.

Bhaskaram, P. & Reddy, V. 1982a. Cutaneous inflammatory response in kwashiorkor. *Indian Journal of Medical Research, 76: 849–853.*

Bhaskaram, P. & Reddy, V. 1982b. Macrophage function in kwashiorkor. *Indian Journal of Pediatrics,* 49: 497–499.

Black, R., Allen, L.H., Bhutta, Z.A., Caufield, L.E., de Onis, M., Ezzati, M., Mathers, C. & Rivera, J. 2008. Maternal and child undernutrition: global and regional exposures and health consequences. *Lancet,* 371(9608): 243–260.

Black, R.E., Victora, C.G., Walker, S.P., Bhutta, Z.A., Christian, P., de Onis, M., Ezzati, M., Grantham-McGregor, S., Katz, J., Martorell, R. & Uauy, R. 2013. Maternal and child undernutrition and overweight in low-income and middle income countries. Paper 1. Lancet Maternal and Child Nutrition Series. *Lancet,* 382(9890): 427–451.

Blaser, M.J. & Newman, L.S. 1982. A review of human salmonellosis: I. Infective dose. *Reviews of Infectious Diseases,* 4(6): 1096–1106.

Boaz, R.T., Joseph, A.J., Kang, G. & Bose, A. 2013. Intestinal permeability in normally nourished and malnourished children with and without diarrhea. *Indian Pediatrics,* 50: 152–153.

Bollaerts, K., Aerts, M., Faes, C., Grijspeerdt, K., Dewulf, J. & Mintiens, K. 2008. Human salmonellosis: estimation of dose-illness from outbreak data. *Risk Analysis,* 28(2): 427–440.

Boring, J.R. III., Martin, W.T. & Elliott, L.M. 1971. Isolation of Salmonella typhimurium from municipal water, Riverside, California, 1965. *American Journal of Epidemiology,* 93: 49–54.

Brent, A.J., Oundo, J.O., Mwangi, I., Ochola, L., Lowe, B. & Berkley, J.A. 2006. Salmonella bacteremia in Kenyan children. *Pediatric Infectious Disease Journal,* 25: 230–236.

Brewster, D.R., Manary, M.J., Menzies, I.S., O'Loughlin, E.V. & Henry, R.L. 1997. Intestinal permeability in kwashiorkor. *Archives of Disease in Childhood,* 76: 236–241.

Bronzan, R.N., Taylor, T.E., Mwenechanya, J., Tembo, M., Kayira, K., Bwanaisa, L., Njobvu, A., Kondowe, W., Chalira, C., Walsh, A.L., Phiri, A., Wilson, L.K., Molyneux, M.E. & Graham, S.M. 2007. Bacteremia in Malawian children with severe malaria: prevalence, etiology, HIV co-infection, and outcome. *Journal of Infectious Diseases,* 195: 895–904.

Buchanan, R.L. & Schaffner, D. 2015. FSMA: Testing as a tool for verifying preventive controls. *Food Protection Trends,* 35: 228–237.

Burnett, S.L., Gehm, E.B., Weissinger, W.R. & Beuchat, L.R. 2000. Survival of Salmonella in peanut butter and peanut spread. *Journal of Applied Microbiology,* 89: 472–477.

Codex Alimentarius Commission (CAC). 1969. *General Principles of Food Hygiene* [CAC/RCP-1/1969]. (also available at www.codexalimentarius.org/download/standards/23/CXP_001e.pdf).

Codex Alimentarius Commission (CAC). 1997. *Principles and Guidelines for the Establishment and Application of Microbiological Criteria Related to Foods* [CAC/GL-21]. (also available at www.codexalimentarius.org/download/standards/394/CXG_021e.pdf).

Codex Alimentarius Commission (CAC). 2015. *Code of Hygienic Practice for Low-moisture Foods.* [CAC/RCP-75/2015]. (also available at www.codexalimentarius.org/download/standards/13921/CXP_075e_2015.pdf).

Carvalho Neves Forte, W., Martins Campos, J.V. & Carneiro Leao, R. 1984. Non specific immunological response in moderate malnutrition. *Allergologia et immunopathologia,* 12: 489–496.

Castillo-Duran, C., Heresi, G., Fisberg, M. & Uauy, R. 1987. Controlled trial of zinc supplementation during recovery from malnutrition: effects on growth and immune function. *American Journal of Clinical Nutrition,* 45: 602–608.

Cavallaro, E., Date, K., Medus, C., Meyer, S., Miller, B., Kim, C., Nowicki, S., Cosgrove, S., Sweat, D., Phan, Q., Flint, J., Daly, E.R., Adams, J., Hyytia-Trees, E., Gerner-Smidt, P., Hoekstra, R.M., Schwensohn, C., Langer, A., Sodha, S.V., Rogers, M.C., Angulo, F.J., Tauxe, R.V., Williams, I.T., Behravesh, C.B. & Salmonella Typhimurium Outbreak Investigation Team. 2011. Salmonella typhimurium infections associated with peanut products. *New England Journal of Medicine,* 365(7): 601–610.

Centers for Disease Control and Prevention (CDC). 2009. Multistate outbreak of Salmonella typhimurium infections linked to peanut butter, 2008–2009 (Final Update). In: *CDC* [online]. [Cited 15 October 2015]. www.cdc.gov/salmonella/2009/peanut-butter-2008-2009.html

Chevalier, P. 1997. Thymic ultrasonography in children, a non-invasive assessment of nutritional immune deficiency. *Nutrition Research,* 17: 1271–1276.

Chevalier, P., Sevilla, R., Sejas, E., Zalles, L., Belmonte, G. & Parent, G. 1998. Immune recovery of malnourished children takes longer than nutritional recovery: implications for treatment and discharge. *Journal of Tropical Pediatrics,* 44: 304–307.

Chevalier, P., Sevilla, R., Zalles, L., Sejas, E., Belmonte, G. & Parent, G. 1994. Study of thymus and thymocytes in Bolivian preschool children during recovery from severe acute malnutrition. *Journal of Nutrition and Immunology,* 3: 27–39.

Chhangani, L., Sharma, M.L., Sharma, U.B. & Joshi, N. 1985. *In vitro* study of phagocytic and bactericidal activity of neutrophils in cases of protein energy malnutrition. *Indian Journal of Pathology & Microbiology,* 28: 199–203.

Collinson, A.C., Moore, S.E., Cole, T.J. & Prentice, A.M. 2003. Birth season and environmental influences on patterns of thymic growth in rural Gambian infants. *Acta Paediatrica,* 92: 1014–1020.

Craven, P.C., Mackel, D.C., Baine, W.B., Barker, W.H. & Gangarosa, E.J. 1975. International outbreak of Salmonella eastbourne infection traced to contaminated chocolate. *The Lancet,* 1(7910): 788–792.

Crump, J.A., Medalla, F.M., Joyce, K.W., Krueger, A.L., Hoekstra, R.M., Whichard, J.M. & Barzilay, E.J. 2011. Emerging Infections Program NARMS Working Group. Antimicrobial resistance among invasive non-typhoidal *Salmonella enterica* isolates in the United States: National Antimicrobial Resistance Monitoring System, 1996 to 2007. Antimicrobial Agents and Chemotherapy, 55(3): 1148–1154.

D'Aoust, J.Y. 1985. Infective dose of Salmonella typhimurium in cheddar cheese. *American Journal of Epidemiology,* 122(4): 717–720.

D'Aoust, J.Y., Aris, B.J., Thisdele, P., Durante, A., Brisson, N., Dragon, D., Lachapelle, G., Johnston, M. & Laidely, R. 1975. *Salmonella* eastbourne outbreak associated with chocolate. *Journal Institut Canadien de Technologie Alimentaire,* 8: 181–184.

Douglas, S.D. & Schopfer, K. 1974. Phagocyte function in protein-calorie malnutrition. *Clinical and Experimental Immunology,* 17: 121–128.

Edelman, R. 1973. Cutaneous hypersensitivity in protein-calorie malnutrition. *Lancet,* 1(7814): 1244–1245.

Fakhir, S., Ahmad, P., Faridi, M.A. & Rattan, A. 1989. Cell-mediated immune responses in malnourished host. *Journal of Tropical Pediatrics,* 35: 175–178.

FAO & WHO. 2002. Hazard characterization of *Salmonella. In: Risk assessment of* Salmonella *in eggs and broiler chickens,* pp. 17–96. Microbiological Risk Assessment Series No. 2. Rome. 301 pp. (also available at www.fao.org/3/a-y4392e.pdf).

FAO & WHO. 2003. *Hazard characterization for pathogens in food and water.* Microbiological Risk Assessment Series No. 3. Rome. 31 p. (also available at www.fao.org/3/a-y4666e.pdf).

FAO & WHO. 2016a. *Microbial safety of lipid-based ready-to-use food for management of moderate acute malnutrition and severe acute malnutrition.* First report. Report of 2012 expert meeting. Microbiological Risk Assessment Series No. 28. Rome. 80 pp. (also available at www.fao.org/3/a-i5347e.pdf).

FAO & WHO. 2016b. *Statistical aspects of microbiological criteria related to foods: a risk manager's guide.* Microbiological Risk Assessment Series No. 24. Rome. 120 pp. (also available at www.fao.org/3/a-i3996e.pdf).

Fazil, A.M. 1996. *A quantitative risk assessment model for* Salmonella. Drexel University. (Dissertation)

Feasey, N.A., Dougan, G., Kingsley, R.A., Heydermans, R.S. & Gordan, M.A. 2012. Invasive non-typhoidal salmonella disease: an emerging and neglected tropical disease in Africa. *Lancet,* 379(9835): 2489–2499.

Fernandez, I.D., Himes, J.H. & De Onis, M. 2001. Prevalence of nutritional wasting in populations: building explanatory models using secondary data. *Bulletin of the World Health Organization,* 80(4): 282–291.

Fongwo, N.P., Arinola, O.G. & Salimonu, L.S. 1999. Leucocyte migration inhibition factor (L-MIF) in malnourished Nigerian children. *African Journal of Medicine and Medical Sciences,* 28: 17–20.

Fontaine, R.E., Cohen, M.L., Martin, W.T. & Vernon, T.M. 1980. Epidemic salmonellosis from cheddar cheese: Surveillance and Prevention. *American Journal of Epidemiology,* 111: 247–253.

Fontaine, R.E., Arnon, S., Martin, W.T., Vernon, T.M. Jr., Gangarosa, E.J., Farmer, J.J. III., Moran, A.B., Silliker, J.H. & Decker, D.L. 1978. Raw hamburger: an interstate common source of human salmonellosis. *American Journal of Epidemiology,* 107: 36–45.

Forsythe, S.J., Dickins, B. & Jolley, K.A. 2014. *Cronobacter,* the emergent bacterial pathogen *Enterobacter sakazakii* comes of age; MLST and whole genome sequence analysis. *BMC Genomics,* 15: 11–21.

Garly, M.L., Trautner, S.L., Marx, C., Danebod, K., Nielsen, J., Ravn, H., Martins, C.L., Bale, C., Aaby, P. & Lisse, I.M. 2008. Thymus size at 6 months of age and subsequent child mortality. *Journal of Pediatrics,* 153(5): 683–688.

Geefhuysen, J., Rosen, E.U., Katz, J., Ipp, T. & Metz, J. 1971. Impaired cellular immunity in kwashiorkor with improvement after therapy. *British Medical Journal,* 4: 527–529.

George, R.H. 1976. Small infectious doses of *Salmonella. Lancet,* 1(7969): 1130–1130.

Glynn, J.R. & Bradley, D.J. 1992. The relationship between infecting dose and severity of disease in reported outbreaks of *Salmonella* infections. *Epidemiology and Infection,* 109(3): 371–388.

Goyal, H.K., Kaushik, S.K., Dhamieja, J.P., Suman, R.K. & Kumar, K.K. 1981. A study of granulocyte adherence in protein calorie malnutrition. *Indian Pediatrics,* 18: 287–292.

Graham, S.M. 2010. Non-typhoidal salmonellosis in Africa. *Current Opinions in Infectious Diseases,* 23: 409–414.

Gray, N., Bedford, J., Deconinck, H. & Brown, R. (CMAM Forum and Anthrologica). 2014. *Community Engagement the 'C' at the heart of CMAM.* CMAM Forum Technical Brief.

Green, F. & Heyworth, B. 1980. Immunoglobulin-containing cells in jejunal mucosa of children with protein-energy malnutrition and gastroenteritis. *Archives of Disease in Childhood,* 55: 380–383.

Greenwood, B.M., Bradley-Moore, A.M., Bradley, A.K., Kirkwood, B.R. & Gilles, H.M. 1986. The immune response to vaccination in undernourished and well-nourished Nigerian children. *Annals of Tropical Medicine and Parasitology,* 80: 537–544.

Greenwood, M.H. & Hooper, W.L. 1983. Chocolate bars contaminated with Salmonella napoli: an infectivity study. *British Medical Journal,* 286: 1394.

Grocery Manufacturers Association (GMA). 2009. *Control of Salmonella in low-moisture foods.* https://forms.consumerbrandsassociation.org//forms/store/ProductFormPublic/SalmonellaControlGuidance.

Harland, P.S. 1965. Tuberculin reactions in malnourished children. *Lancet,* 2: 719–721.

Hennessy, T.W., Hedberg, C.W., Slutsker, L., White, K., Besser-Wiek, J.M., Moen, E., Feldman, J., Coleman, W.W., Edmonson, L.M., MacDonald, K.L. & Osterholm, M.T. 1966. A national outbreak of *Salmonella enteritidis* infections from ice cream. *New England Journal of Medicine,* 334(20): 1281–1286.

Heyworth, B. 1977. Delayed hypersensitivity to PPD-S following BCG vaccination in African children–an 18-month field study. *Transactions of the Royal Society of Tropical Medicine and Hygiene,* 71: 251–253.

Hohmann. E.L. 2015. Non-typhoidal *Salmonella* bacteremia [online]. In: *UpToDate.* [Cited 27 June 2015]. www.uptodate.com/contents/nontyphoidal-salmonella-bacteremia.

Holy, O. & Forsythe, S.J. 2014. *Cronobacter* species as emerging causes of healthcare-associated infection. *Journal of Hospital Infections,* 86: 169–177.

Hossain, M.I., Nahar, B., Hamadani, J.D., Ahmed, T., Roy, A.K. & Brown, K.H. 2010. Intestinal mucosal permeability of severely underweight and non-malnourished Bangladeshi children and effects of nutritional rehabilitation. *Journal of Pediatric Gastroenterology and Nutrition* 51: 638–644.

Hughes, S.M., Amadi, B., Mwiya, M., Nkamba, H., Tomkins, A. & Goldblatt, D. 2009. Dendritic cell anergy results from endotoxaemia in severe malnutrition. *Journal of Immunology,* 183: 2818–2826.

International Commission on Microbiological Specifications for Foods (ICMSF). 2002. *Microbiologic testing in food safety management.* Microorganisms in Foods 7. Springer Science.

International Commission on Microbiological Specifications for Foods (ICMSF). 2011. *Use of data for assessing process control and product acceptance.* Microorganisms in Foods 8. Springer Science.

Jambon, B., Ziegler, O., Maire, B., Hutin, M.F., Parent, G., Fall, M., Burnel, D. & Duheille, J. 1988. Thymulin (facteur thymique serique) and zinc contents of the thymus glands of malnourished children. *American Journal of Clinical Nutrition,* 48: 335–342.

Kasuga, F., Hirota, M., Wada, M., Yunokawa, T., Toyofuku, H., Shibatsuji, M., Michino, H., Kuwasaki, T., Yamamoto, S. & Kumagai, S. 2004. Archiving of food samples from restaurants and caterers—quantitative profiling of outbreaks of foodborne salmonellosis in Japan. *Journal of Food Protection,* 67: 2024–2032.

Keller, S.E., VanDoren, J., Grasso, E.M. & Halik, L.A. 2013. Growth and survival of *Salmonella* in ground black pepper *(Piper nigrum).* Food Microbiology, 34: 182–188.

Keusch, G., Urrutia, J., Guerrero, O., Casteneda, G. & Douglas, S. 1977a. Rosette-forming lymphocytes in Guatemalan children with protein-calorie malnutrition. In R.M. Suskind, ed. *Malnutrition and the Immune Response.* New York, USA, Raven Press.

Keusch, G., Urrutia, J.J., Fernandez, R., Guerrero, O. & Casteneda, G. 1977b. Humoral and cellular aspects of intracellular bactericidal killing in Guatemalan children with protein-energy malnutrition. In R.M. Suskind, ed. *Malnutrition and the Immune Response,* pp. 245–251. New York, USA, Raven Press.

Kielman, A. 1977. Nutritional and immune responses of subclinically malnourished Indian children. In R.M. Suskind, ed. *Malnutrition and the Immune Response.* pp. 429–440. New York, USA, Raven Press.

Kosek, M., Bern, C. & Guerrant, R.L. 2003. The global burden of diarrhoeal disease, as estimated from studies published between 1992 and 2000. *Bulletin of the World Health Organization,* 81: 197–204.

Lagendorf, C., Le Hello, S, Moumouni, A., Gouali, M., Mamaty, A.A., Grasi, R.F., Weill, F.-X. & Page, A.-L. 2015. Enteric bacterial pathogens in children with diarrhea in Niger: Diversity and antimicrobial resistance. *PLOS One,* 3: e0120275 [online]. [Cited 27 June 2015]. https://journals.plos.org/plosone/article?id=10.1371/journal.pone.0120275

Lehmacher, A., Bockemuhl, J. & Aleksic, S. 1995. Nationwide outbreak of human salmonellosis in Germany due to contaminated paprika and paprika-powdered potato chips. *Epidemiology and Infection,* 115: 501–511.

Leitzmann, C., Vithayasai, V., Windecker, P., Suskind, R. & Olson, R. 1977. Phagocytosis and killing function of polymorphnuclear leukocytes in Thai children with protein-energy malnutrition. In R.M. Suskind, ed. *Malnutrition and the Immune Response,* pp. 253–257. New York, USA, Raven Press.

Lima, A.A.M., Fang, G.D., Schorling, J.B., Dealbuquerque, L., McAuliffe, J.F., Mota, S., Leite, R. & Guerrant, R.L. 1992. Persistent diarrhea in Northeast Brazil – etiologies and interactions with malnutrition. *Acta Paediatrica,* 81(Suppl. 381): 39–44.

Lipson, M. 1976. Infecting dose of *Salmonella. Lancet,* 969.

Lotfy, O.A., Saleh, W.A. & el-Barbari, M. 1998. A study of some changes of cell-mediated immunity in protein energy malnutrition. *Journal of the Egyptian Society of Parasitology,* 28: 413–428.

Machado, R.M., da Costa, J.C., de Lima Filho, E.C., Brasil, M.R. & da Rocha, G.M. 1985. Longitudinal study of the nitroblue tetrazolium test in children with protein-calorie malnutrition. *Journal of Tropical Pediatrics,* 31: 74–77.

Majowicz, S.E., Musto, J., Scallan, E., Angulo, F.J., Kirk, M., O'Brian, S.J., Jones, T.F., Fazil, A. & Hoekstra, R.M. 2010. The global burden of non-typhoidal salmonella gastro-enteritis. *Clinical Infectious Disease,* 50(6): 882–889.

Matsui, T., Suzuki, S., Takahashi, H., Ohyama, T., Kobayashi, J., Izumiya, H., Watanabe, H., Kasuga, F., Kijima, H., Shibata, K. &, Okabe, N. 2004. *Salmonella* Enteritidis outbreak associated with a school-lunch dessert: cross-contamination and a long incubation period, Japan, 2001 *Epidemiology and Infection,* 132: 873–879.

McMurray, D.N., Watson, R.R. & Reyes, M.A. 1981. Effect of re-nutrition on humoral and cell-mediated immunity in severely malnourished children. *American Journal of Clinical Nutrition,* 34: 2117–2126.

McMurray, D.N., Loomis, S.A., Casazza, L.J., Rey, H. & Miranda, R. 1981. Development of impaired cell-mediated immunity in mild and moderate malnutrition. *American Journal of Clinical Nutrition, 34: 68–77.*

Ministry of Health and Welfare, Japan. 1999. Research on microbiological risk assessment, prepared by Susumu Kumagai and Shigeki Yamamoto. In: *Report of Grants for Health Science of the Ministry of Health and Welfare, Japan.*

Moore, S.E., Prentice, A.M., Wagatsuma, Y., Fulford, A.J., Collinson, A.C., Raqib, R., Vahter, M., Persson, L.A. & Arifeen, S.E. 2009. Early-life nutritional and environmental determinants of thymic size in infants born in rural Bangladesh. *Acta Paediatrica,* 98: 1168–1175.

Naeye, R.L. 1965. Organ and cellular development in congenital heart disease and in alimentary malnutrition. *Journal of Pediatrics,* 67: 447–458.

Najera, O., Gonzalez, C., Cortes, E., Toledo, G. & Ortiz, R. 2004. Flow cytometry study of lymphocyte subsets in malnourished and well-nourished children with bacterial infections. *Clinical and Diagnostic Laboratory Immunology,* 11: 577–580.

Najera, O., Gonzalez, C., Cortes, E., Toledo, G. & Ortiz, R. 2007. Effector T lymphocytes in well-nourished and malnourished infected children. *Clinical and Experimental Immunology,* 148: 501–506.

Najera, O., Gonzalez, C., Toledo, G., Lopez, L., Cortes, E., Betancourt, M. & Ortiz, R. 2001. CD45RA and CD45RO isoforms in infected malnourished and infected well-nourished children. *Clinical and Experimental Immunology,* 126:461-465.

Nassar, M.F., El-Batrawy, S.R., Nagy, N.M. 2009. CD95 expression in white blood cells of malnourished infants during hospitalization and catch-up growth. *Eastern Mediterranean Health Journal,* 15: 574–583.

Nassar, M.F., Younis, N.T., Tohamy, A.G., Dalam, D.M. & El Badawy, M.A. 2007. T-lymphocyte subsets and thymic size in malnourished infants in Egypt: a hospital-based study. *Eastern Mediterranean Health Journal,* 13: 1031–1042.

Norton, E.B., Archibald, L.K., Nwanyanwu, O.C., Kazembe, P.N., Dobbie, H., Reller, L.B., Jarvis, W.R. & Jason, J. 2004. Clinical predictors of bloodstream infections and mortality in hospitalized Malawian children. *Pediatric Infectious Disease Journal,* 23(2): 145–151; discussion pp. 151–155.

Page, A.-L., de Rekeneire, N., Sayadi, S., Aberrane, S, Janssens, A.-C., Reiux, C., Djibo, A., Manuguerra, J-C., Ducou-le-Pointe, H., Grais, R.F., Scjarefer, M., Geurin, P.J. & Baron, E. 2013. Infections in children admitted with complicated severe acute malnutrition in Niger. *PLOS One,* vol. 8: e68699 [online]. [Cited 27 June 2015]. https://journals.plos.org/plosone/article?id=10.1371/journal.pone.0068699

Parent, G., Chevalier, P., Zalles, L., Sevilla, R., Bustos, M., Dhenin, J.M. & Jambon, B. 1994. *In vitro* lymphocyte-differentiating effects of thymulin (Zn-FTS) on lymphocyte subpopulations of severely malnourished children. *American Journal of Clinical Nutrition,* 60: 274–278.

Patwari, A. 1999. Diarrhoea and malnutrition interaction. *Indian Journal of Pediatrics,* 66(Suppl.): S124–134.

Picot, J., Hartwell, D., Harris, P., Mendes, D., Clegg, A.J. & Takeda, A. 2012. The effectiveness of interventions to treat severe acute malnutrition in your children: a systematic review. *Health Technology Assessment, 16(19): 1*–316.

Podolak, R., Enache, E., Sonte, W., Black, D.G. & Elliott, P.H. 2010. Sources and risk factors for contamination, survival, persistence, and heat resistance of *Salmonella* in low-moisture foods. *Journal of Food Protection,* 73: 1919–1936.

Proaña Peralta, L.G., Friedrich, L.M., Harris, L.J. & Danyluk, M.D. 2011. Survival of *Salmonella* spp., *Listeria monocytogenes* and *Escherichia coli* O157:H7 on inoculated peanut and pecan kernels stored at -20°C, 4°C and 23°C. *Journal of Food Protection,* 74(Suppl. A): 199.

Puri, V., Misra, P.K., Saxena, K.C., Saxsena, P.N., Saxena, R.P. & Agarwal, C.G. 1980. Immune status in malnutrition. *Indian Pediatrics,* 17: 127–133.

Purtilo, D.T., Riggs, R.S., Evans, R. & Neafie, R.C. 1976. Humoral immunity of parasitized, malnourished children. *American Journal of Tropical Medicine and Hygiene,* 25: 229–232.

Raman, T.S. 1992. Nitroblue tetrazolium test in protein energy malnutrition. *Indian Pediatrics,* 29: 355–356.

Reddy, V., Raghuramulu, N. & Bhaskaram, C. 1976. Secretory IgA in protein-calorie malnutrition. *Archives of Disease in Childhood,* 51: 871–874.

Reddy, V., Jagadeesan, V., Ragharamulu, N., Bhaskaram, C. & Srikantia, S.G. 1976. Functional significance of growth retardation in malnutrition. *American Journal of Clinical Nutrition,* 29: 3–7.

Rich, K., Neumann, C. & Stiehm, R. 1977. Neutrophil chemotaxis in malnourished Ghanaian children. In R.M. Suskind, ed. *Malnutrition and the Immune Response,* pp. 271–275. New York, USA, Raven Press.

Rikimaru, T., Taniguchi, K., Yartey, J.E., Kennedy, D.O. & Nkrumah, F.K. 1998. Humoral and cell-mediated immunity in malnourished children in Ghana. *European Journal of Clinical Nutrition,* 52: 344–350.

Rosen, E.U., Geefhuysen, J., Anderson, R., Joffe, M. & Rabson, A.R. 1975. Leucocyte function in children with kwashiorkor. *Archives of Disease in Childhood,* 50: 220–224.

Ross, T., Fratamico, P., Jaykus, L.A. Zwietering, M. 2011. Statistics of sampling for microbiological testing of foodborne pathogens. In J. Hoorfar, ed. *Rapid detection, characterization, and enumeration of food-borne pathogens,* pp. 103–120. Washington, USA, ASM Press.

Rytter, M.J., Kolte, L., Briend, A., Friis, H. & Christensen, V.B. 2014. The immune system in children with malnutrition–a systematic review. *PLOS One,* vol. 9: e105017 [online]. [Cited 27 June 2015]. https://journals.plos.org/plosone/article?id=10.1371/journal.pone.0105017

Sakamoto, M. & Nishioka, K. 1992. Complement system in nutritional deficiency. *World Review of Nutrition and Dietetics,* 67: 114–139.

Salimonu, L.S., Ojo-Amaize, E., Johnson, A.O., Laditan, A.A., Akinwolere, O.A. & Wigzell, H. 1983. Depressed natural killer cell activity in children with protein-calorie malnutrition. II. Correction of the impaired activity after nutritional recovery. *Cellular Immunology*, 82: 210–215.

Salimonu, L.S., Ojo-Amaize, E., Williams, A.I., Johnson, A.O., Cooke, A.R., Adekunle, F.A., Alm, G.V. & Wigzell, H. 1982. Depressed natural killer cell activity in children with protein-calorie malnutrition. *Clinical Immunology and Immunopathology*, 24: 1–7.

Santillana Farakos, S.M., Frank, J.F. & Schaffner, D.W. 2013. Modelling the influence of temperature, water activity and water mobility on the persistence of *Salmonella* in low-moisture foods. *International Journal of Food Microbiology*, 166: 280–293.

Satyanarayana, K., Bhaskaram, P., Seshu, V.C. & Reddy, V. 1980. Influence of nutrition on postvaccinial tuberculin sensitivity. *American Journal of Clinical Nutrition*, 33: 2334–2337.

Savy, M., Edmond, K., Fine, P.E., Hall, A., Hennig, B.J., Moore, S.E., Mulholland, K., Schaible. U. & Prentice, A.M. 2009. Landscape analysis of interactions between nutrition and vaccine responses in children. *Journal of Nutrition*, 139: 2154S–2218S

Scallan, E., Hoekstra, R.M., Angulo, F.J., Tauxe, R.V., Widdowson, M.-A., Roy, S.L., Jones, J.L. & Griffin, P.M. 2011. Foodborne illness acquired in the United States – Major pathogens. *Emerging Infectious Diseases*, 17(1): 7–15.

Scallan, E., Majowicz, S.E., Hall, G., Banerjee, A., Bowman, C.L., Daly, L., Jones, T. Kirk, M.D., Fitzgerald, M. & Angulo, F.J. 2005. Prevalence of diarrhoea in the community in Australia, Canada, Ireland and the United States. *International Journal of Epidemiology*, 34: 454–460.

Schlesinger, L. & Stekel, A. 1974. Impaired cellular immunity in marasmic infants. *American Journal of Clinical Nutrition*, 27: 615–620.

Schonland, M. 1972. Depression of immunity in protein-calorie malnutrition: a post-mortem study. *Journal of Tropical Pediatrics and Environmental Child Health*, 18: 217–224.

Schopfer, K. & Douglas, S.D. 1976a. Fine structural studies of peripheral blood leucocytes from children with kwashiorkor: morphological and functional properties. *British Journal of Haematology*, 32: 573–577.

Schopfer, K. & Douglas, S.D. 1976b. Neutrophil function in children with kwashiorkor. *Journal of Laboratory and Clinical Medicine*, 88: 450–461.

Seth, V., Kukreja, N., Sundaram, K.R. & Malaviya, A.N. 1981. Delayed hypersensitivity after BCG in pre-school children in relation to their nutritional status. *Indian Journal of Medical Research*, 74: 392–398.

Shilotri, P.G. 1976. Hydrogen peroxide production by leukocytes in protein-calorie malnutrition. *Clinica Chimica Acta – International Journal of Clinical Chemistry,* 71: 511–514.

Shiner, M., Redmond, A.O. & Hansen, J.D. 1973. The jejunal mucosa in protein-energy malnutrition. A clinical, histological, and ultra-structural study. *Experimental and Molecular Pathology,* 19: 61–78.

Shousha, S. & Kamel, K. 1972. Nitro blue tetrazolium test in children with kwashiorkor with a comment on the use of latex particles in the test. *Journal of Clinical Pathology,* 25: 494–497.

Smith, N., Khadroui, S., Lopez, V. & Hamza, B. 1977. Cellular immune response in Tunisian children with severe infantile malnutrition. In R.M. Suskind, ed. *Malnutrition and the Immune Response.* New York, USA, Raven Press.

Smythe, P.M., Brereton-Stiles, G.G., Grace, H.J., Mafoyane, A., Schonland, M., Coovadia, H.M., Loening, W.E., Parent, M.A. & Vos, G.H. 1971. Thymolymphatic deficiency and depression of cell-mediated immunity in protein-calorie malnutrition. *Lancet,* 2: 939–943.

Stanfield, J.P., Hutt, M.S. & Tunnicliffe, R. 1965. Intestinal biopsy in kwashiorkor. *Lancet,* 2: 519–523.

Sullivan, P.B., Lunn, P.G., Northrop-Clewes, C., Crowe, P.T., Marsh, M.N. Neale, G. 1992. Persistent diarrhea and malnutrition–the impact of treatment on small bowel structure and permeability. *Journal of Pediatric Gastroenterology and Nutrition,* 14: 208–215.

Tejada, C., Argueta, V., Sanchez, M. & Albertazzi, C. 1964. Phagocytic and alkaline phosphatase activity of leukocytes in kwashiorkor. *Journal of Pediatrics,* 64: 753–761.

Teunis, P.F., Kasuga, F., Fazil, A., Ogden, I.D., Rotariu, O. & Strachan, N.J. 2010. Dose-response modelling of *Salmonella* using outbreak data. *International Journal of Food Microbiology,* 144: 243–249.

Theron, J.J., Wittmann, W. & Prinsloo, J.G. 1971. The fine structure of the jejunum in kwashiorkor. *Experimental and Molecular Pathology,* 14: 184–199.

Trehan, I., Goldbach, H.S., LaGrone, L.N., Meuli, G.J., Wang, R.J., Maleta, K.M. & Manary, M.J. 2013. Antibiotics as part of the management of severe acute malnutrition. *New England Journal of Medicine,* 368: 425–435.

UNICEF, WHO & World Bank. 2015. Joint child malnutrition estimates. In: *World Bank* [online]. [Cited 15 May 2015]. http://data.worldbank.org/child-malnutrition

van Schothorst, M., Zwietering, M.H., Ross, T., Buchanan, R.L, Cole, M.B. & International Commission on Microbiological Specifications for Foods. 2009. Relating microbiological criteria to food safety objectives and performance objectives. *Food Control,* 20: 967–979.

Vasquez-Garibay, E., Mendez-Estrada, C., Romero-Velarde, E., Garcia-Iglesias, M.T. & Campollo-Rivas, O. 2004. Nutritional support with nucleotide addition favors immune response in severely malnourished infants. *Archives of Medical Research,* 35: 284–288.

Vasquez-Garibay, E., Campollo-Rivas, O., Romero-Velarde, E., Mendez-Estrada, C., Garcia-Iglesias, T., Alvizo-Mora, J.G. & Vizmanos-Lamotte, B. 2002. Effect of re-nutrition on natural and cell-mediated immune response in infants with severe malnutrition. *Journal of Pediatric Gastroenterology and Nutrition,* 34: 296–301.

Vought, K.J. & Tatini, S.R. 1998. *Salmonella* enteritidis contamination of ice cream associated with a 1994 multistate outbreak. *Journal of Food Protection,* 61: 5–10.

Watts, T. 1969. Thymus weights in malnourished children. *Journal of Tropical Pediatrics,* 15: 155–158.

WHO. 2012. *Technical note: supplementary foods for the management of moderate acute malnutrition in infants and children 6–59 months of age.* Geneva.

WHO. 2013a. *Guideline: Updates on the management of severe acute malnutrition in infants and children.* 44 pp.

WHO. 2013b. *Diarrhoeal disease.* https://www.who.int/news-room/fact-sheets/detail/diarrhoeal-disease#:~:text=Scope%20of%20diarrhoeal%20disease&text=In%20low%2Dincome%20countries%2C%20children,episodes%20of%20diarrhoea%20every%20year.

World Health Organization, World Food Programme, United Nations System Standing Committee on Nutrition & United Nations Children's Fund (WHO, WFP, UNSCN & UNICEF). 2007. *Community-based management of severe acute malnutrition.* A Joint Statement by WHO, WFP, UNSCN and UNICEF.

Wolfsdorf, J. & Nolan, R. 1974. Leucocyte function in protein deficiency states. *South African Medical Journal,* 48: 528–530.

Ziegler, H.D. & Ziegler, P.B. 1975. Depression of tuberculin reaction in mild and moderate protein-calorie malnourished children following BCG vaccination. *Johns Hopkins Medical Journal,* 137: 59–64.

Annexes

Annex 1

Overview of ready-to-use foods for acute malnutrition

Objective	Treatment of severe acute malnutrition (SAM)	Treatment of moderate acute malnutrition (MAM)
Generic Term	Ready-to-use therapeutic foods	Ready-to-use supplementary foods
	(RUTFs)	(RUSFs)
		High quantity (92 g)
Products	imunut, Plumpy Nut, eeZeePaste and VN,	eeZeeRUSF and Plumpy Sup
Purpose	Treatment of uncomplicated SAM with continued breastfeeding. SAM is defined as presence of nutritional oedema or mid-upper arm circumference (MUAC) < 115 mm or weight for height < -3Z by WHO 2006 growth tables	Supplement to manage MAM with continued breastfeeding. MAM is defined as MUAC 115–124 mm or weight-for-height Z score between 3Z and 2Z according to WHO 2006 growth tables
Target group	Infants and children 6–59 months with uncomplicated SAM; and older patients with SAM	Infants and children 6–59 months with WFH between 3Z and 2Z or MUAC < 125 mm
	Children may transition from F75/F100 in hospital settings to RUTF adults including those with HIV	Others such as HIV-positive adults, pregnant a lactating women
	May also be used as convalescent feeding, for example 2 weeks ration following episode of measles or malaria	May also be used as convalescent feeding, for example 2 weeks ration following episode of measles or malaria
Directions for use	Eaten directly from sachet, without dilution or cooking; drinking water must be available Indicated on the individual packaging	Eaten directly from sachet, without dilution or cooking; Indicated on the individual packaging

	Micronutrient and chronic malnutrition prevention		
y-to-use supplementary ;	Lipid-based nutrient supplements	Lipid-based nutrient supplements	Lipid-based nutrient supplements (LNS)
Fs)	(LNS)	(LNS)	*Low quantity (20 g)*
quantity (100 g)	*Medium quantity (50 g)*	*Medium quantity (46 g)*	
Mum	Wawa Mum	Plumpy Doz and eeZeeCup	Nutributter
'ement to manage MAM :ontinued breastfeeding	Supplement the local diet for prevention of acute malnutrition with continued breastfeeding and prevent micronutrient deficiency and stunting	Supplement to the local diet for prevention of acute malnutrition with continued breastfeeding and prevent micronutrient deficiency and stunting	Supplement to the local diet with continued breastfeeding to prevent micronutrient deficiency and stunting
ts and children 6–59 months WFH between 3Z and 2Z or : < 125 mm	Infants and children 6–23 months	Infants and children 6–23 months	Infants and babies 6–23 months
directly from sachet, ut dilution or cooking; ted on the individual ging	Eaten directly from sachet, without dilution or cooking; Indicated on the individual packaging	Eaten directly from sachet, without dilution or cooking; Indicated on the individual packaging	Eaten directly from sachet, without dilution or cooking; Indicated on the individual packaging

(cont.)

Objective	Treatment of severe acute malnutrition (SAM)	Treatment of moderate acute malnutrition (MAM)
Sole source of food	Yes (100% of daily energy and micronutrient requirements)	No (generally 25–50% of daily energy and up to 10 of micronutrient requirements)
Ingredients	Sugar, vegetable oil (palm, soybean, canola),peanuts or peanut paste, skimmed milked, whole milk or whey powders, vitamin and mineral pre-mix, stabilizer (hydrogenated fat), emulsifier (mono- or di-glycerides)	Vegetable fats, sugar, peanut paste, soybean proteins, maltodextrin and whey, vitamin and mineral complex
Energy/ nutrients per 100 g	520–550 kcal	500 kcal
	12.5 g protein	12.5 g protein
	32.9 g fat	32.9 g fat
	65 g carbohydrate	65 g carbohydrate
	Moisture 2.5% (A_w = 0.6%)	Moisture 2.5% (A_w = 0.6%)
	Vitamin and mineral pre-mix: vitamin A, B1, B2, B3, B5, B6, folic acid, vitamin C, D, E, K. Minerals Na, K, Ca, P, Mg, Fe (10–14 mg) Zn (10 mg),Cu, Se, I	Vitamin and mineral pre-mix: vitamin A, B1, B2, B3, B5, B6, folic acid, vitamin C, D, E, K. Minera Na, K, Ca, P, Mg, Fe, Zn, Cu, Se, I
Packaging	1 Sachet = 92 g printed aluminium foil sachet; often nitrogen flushed	Sachet = 92 g printed aluminium foil; sachet; c nitrogen flushed
Shelf life	24 months from manufacturing date	24 months from manufacturing date
Ration/dose	According to weight:	One sachet per day about 92 g/day (about 75 kcal/kg/day)
	6–59 months: 200 kcal/kg/day; in practice: 2–3 sachets/day, or 184–276 g/day	

	Micronutrient and chronic malnutrition prevention		
	No	No	No
kpeas, vegetable oil, med milk powder, sugar, nins (A, B1, B2, B3, B5, B6, 9, B12, C, D, E, K), minerals Cu, I, Fe, Mg, P, K, Zn) and sifier	Chickpeas, vegetable oil, skimmed milk powder, sugar, vitamins (A, B1, B2, B3, B5, B6, B7, B9, B12, C, D, E, K), minerals (Ca, Cu, I, Fe, Mg, P, K, Zn) and emulsifier	Blended vegetable oil (palm, soybean, canola) peanuts, sugar, non-fat milk powder, whey, maltodextrin, vitamin and mineral pre-mix, cocoa, (optional) emulsifier)	Peanut paste, sugar, vegetable oil (palm, soybean, canola), non-fat milk powder, whey, maltodextrin, vitamin and mineral complex, emulsifier, lecithin
kcal	About 240 kcal	247 kcal	108 kcal
protein	6.5 g protein	5.9 g protein	2.5g protein
fat	14.5 g fat	16 g fat	7 g fat
		65 g carbohydrate	65 g carbohydrate
ture 2.5% (A_w = 0.5%)	Moisture 2.5% (A_w = 0.5%)	Moisture 2.5% (A_w = 0.6%)	Moisture 2.5% (A_w = 0.6%)
kcal, 13 g protein (10%), 29 g 0%). Contains EFA, meets nd PDCAAS. Vitamin and ral pre-mix: vitamin A, B1, 3, B5, B6, folic acid, vitamin E, K. Minerals Na, K, Ca, P, Fe, Zn, Cu, Se, I	260 kcal, 6.5 g protein (10%), 14.5 g fat (50%). Contains EFA, meets RNI and PDCAAS	Vitamin and mineral pre-mix: vitamin A, B1, B2, B3, B5, B6, folic acid, vitamin C, D, E, K. Minerals Na, K, Ca, P, Mg, Fe, Zn, Cu, Mn, Se, I	
et = 100 g printed PET et; often nitrogen flushed	Sachet = 100 g printed aluminium foil sachet; often nitrogen flushed	325 g polypropylene pots or sachets of different quantities. Printed aluminium foil sachet or polypropylene tubs	Aluminium and PET sachet = 20 g
nths from manufacturing	6 months from manufacturing date	24 months from manufacturing date	18 months from manufacturing date
0 g/day; doses administered oon and added to meals. r sachet lasts about 1 week	20 g/day		

(cont.)

Objective	Treatment of severe acute malnutrition (SAM)	Treatment of moderate acute malnutrition (MAM)
Approximate duration of intervention	6–8 weeks	1–3 months
Medical consultation	Yes	No
Concomitant medication	Vitamin A (single dose 50 000 IU–200 000 IU depending on age) Amoxicillin 3 times per day for 5–7 days; albendazole/Mebendazole	No, other than an opportunity for deworming a 6 monthly vitamin A supplementation

	Micronutrient and chronic malnutrition prevention		
onths	3-18 months	3-18 months	Up to 18 months
	No	No, unless used in growth promotion programme	No, unless used in growth promotion programme
	No	No	

Annex 2

Analysis of published models for dose-response of *Salmonella* and additional relevant data, including derivation of exponential dose-response models from *Salmonella* outbreaks associated with low-moisture foods

There are a number of mathematical models proposed to describe how the probability of illness varies with the ingested number of cells of a gastrointestinal pathogen. These are described in FAO and WHO (2003). Of those models, the two that have most often been used in microbiological food safety risk assessment studies are the "exponential" model and the "beta-Poisson" model.

The exponential model has the form:

$$P_{\text{illness}} = 1 - e^{(-r \times \text{dose})}$$

Equation A2.1

where "dose" is expressed as the number of cells of the pathogen that are ingested, and *r is a constant that reflects the probability that an individual cell of the target pathogen will cause infection.*

The beta-Poisson model has the form:

$$P_{\text{illness}} = 1 - [1 + (\text{dose})/alpha]^{-beta}$$

Equation A2.2

where "dose" is expressed as the number of cells of the pathogen that are ingested, and *alpha and beta are parameters to be estimated from the data.*

Importantly, because the exponential model has only one parameter requiring estimation from the data, a model can be fitted from a single observation of dose of *Salmonella* ingested and the observed rate (i.e. probability) of infection among consumers exposed to that dose.

For the purposes of direct comparison with existing dose-response models, and limited data available from salmonellosis outbreaks associated with low-moisture foods (LMFs), including peanut butter (Cavallero *et al.*, 2011) and potato crisps

(Lehmacher, Bockemuhl and Aleksic, 1995), a suite of exponential models were derived to summarize those data.

The existing models considered are the FAO/WHO (2002) model, based on 23 sets of outbreak data, and the Teunis *et al.* (2010) model based on 48 sets of outbreak data. The FAO/WHO (2002) model was originally fitted to a beta-Poisson model, while Teunis *et al.* (2010) uses a more complex approach based on a "multilevel statistical framework." Nonetheless, both models enable the calculation of an $ID_{50,}$ or ID[1]. With this single estimate, an analogous exponential dose-response model can be derived by solving Equation A2.1, with the dose value set to the ID_{50} (or ID_1) of the published model, for which $P_{illness}$ is 0.5 (or 0.01), enabling an estimate of '*r*'.

From this analysis of the FAO/WHO (2002) model fitted to the ID_{50}, the predicted probability of illness from one cell is 1 in 14 000,and from the Teunis *et al.* (2010) model fitted to the ID50, the predicted probability of illness from one cell is 1 in 52.

In the Lehmacher, Bockemuhl and Aleksic (1995) paprika outbreak analysis, there were ≥ 420 confirmed cases. The authors also estimated 10 million × 100 g packs of contaminated potato crisps were consumed, which contained between 0.04 CFU and 0.21 CFU *Salmonella*/g, leading to a median estimated dose of 25 cells. This was equated to $P_{illness}$ of 1 in 10 000 from 25 cells ingested. It has also been estimated that only 1 in 29.3 cases of salmonellosis cases are reported and diagnosed (Scallan *et al.*, 2011). Thus, for the purposes of this crude comparison, it was estimated that the actual number of cases was 12 300, among 10 million exposures to an average of 25 cells. These assumptions produce an ID_{50} estimate of about 5 900 cells, and a probability of illness from one cell of 1 in 8 500.

For the 2009 peanut-butter outbreak in the United States of America (CDC, 2009), it was estimated (D. Zink, USFDA, personal communication, 2014) that there were about 380 cases among 10 million exposures (= 3.8/100 000), and that this was similar to two other large, earlier, peanut-butter outbreaks in the country. The number of cases in these outbreaks was estimated from reported cases and included a factor of 29.3 for underreporting, as for the potato-crisps outbreak. The contamination of such products was assumed to be 1 CFU/g, the lower limit of the testing method used, and it was assumed that a serving consisted of 30 g. While it was considered that only a very small proportion of units were contaminated at all, this was not considered for calculations. Accordingly, the resulting dose-response relationship will most likely underestimate the true risk. These assumptions produce an ID50 estimate of about 547 000 cells, and a probability of illness from one cell of 1 in 789 000.

[1] ID1 is the dose that would be expected to cause illness in 1 percent of "average" consumers.

The above results are summarized in Table A2.1, together with a comparison of the results of refitting the FAO/WHO (2002) and Teunis *et al.* (2010) models fitted to either the ID50 or ID1 of the original published models.

TABLE A2.1 Comparison of predictions of exponential dose-response models for probability of enteric salmonellosis derived from outbreaks involving LMF or published models

	Predictions of analogous exponential dose-response models			
	Potato-crisp outbreak (single observation)	**USA peanut-butter outbreak (single observation)**	**FAO/WHO (2002) (published model)**	**Teunis *et al.* (2010) (published model)**
r derived by fitting to ID_{50}	0.0001174	0.00000127	0.0000722	0.0193
ID_{50}	5 900	547 000	9 600[a]	36[a]
ID_1	85	7931	139	0.5
probability of illness from one cell of *Salmonella*	1 in 8 500	1 in 789 000	1 in 14 000	1 in 52
r derived by fitting to ID_1			0.00248	0.0254
ID_{50}			280	27
ID_1			4.061	0.395[1]
probability of illness from one cell of *Salmonella*			1 in 403	1 in 39

[a]Values taken from the publication or calculated from the published model

Those comparisons indicate that the choice of data, model and modelling approach can have a large effect (orders of magnitude) on the estimated probability of infection at low doses. However, it appears that the FAO/WHO (2002) model as published is consistent with estimates derived from the paprika outbreak analysis (Lehmacher, Bockemuhl and Aleksic, 1995) but orders of magnitude different from the Teunis *et al.* (2002) model and a simple exponential model derived from the 2009 peanut-butter outbreak in the United States of America. Fitting the Teunis *et al.* (2002) dataset to a beta-Poisson model produces a model very similar to the FAO/WHO (2002) model at all relevant dose levels (see Annex 3).

Annex 3

Re-analysis of Teunis *et al.* (2010) dataset as a beta-Poisson model and comparison with the FAO/WHO (2002) *Salmonella* dose-response model

Teunis *et al.* (2010) presented an analysis of available dose-vs-probability of infection data. The dataset used in Teunis *et al.* (2010) included many of the observations used to develop the FAO/WHO (2002) model, but extended the database with new observations. The Teunis et al. (2010) model leads to an ID_{50} estimate of 36.3 cells, some 250-fold lower than predicted by the FAO/WHO (2002) model. Even at low doses, the two models generate very different risk estimates. The FAO/WHO model predicts that a single cell of *Salmonella* might cause illness to 1 in 400 consumers so exposed, whereas the Teunis *et al.* (2010) model infers that the probability of infection from ingestion of a single cell is approximately tenfold greater.[2]

The database upon which the Teunis et al. (2010) model was developed was presented in full in that paper. Teunis *et al.* (2010) used a sophisticated modelling approach, developing models for infection and illness-given-infection using a "multilevel statistical framework." These models incorporated potential differences in pathogen virulence and susceptibility, and adjustments for heterogeneity in exposure. However, the resultant models are complex, and difficult to compare directly with existing models developed using the more established "exponential" or "beta-Poisson" models (FAO and WHO, 2003). Notably, the Teunis *et al.* (2010) approach taken leads to ID_{50} estimates that are orders of magnitude **lower** than expected based on current expert opinion, leading to much higher estimates of risk. The validity of the predictions of the Teunis *et al.* (2010) modelling approach cannot be evaluated because there are insufficient independent observations.

To enable an appreciation of the effects of the model on the predicted probability of infection for different doses, the Teunis *et al.* (2010) dataset was fitted to a beta-Poisson model:

$$P_{illness} = 1 - [1+(dose)/alpha]^{-beta}$$

where "dose" is expressed as the number of cells of the pathogen that are ingested, and *alpha and beta are parameters to be estimated from the data*

2 This estimate was based on the ID1 (dose expected to cause illness in 1 percent of the population) for both models, which is 0.395 for the Teunis *et al.* (2010) model, and 4.1 cells for the FAO/WHO (2002) model.

The model was fitted to the data using two different stochastic assumptions. In the first, the $\log_{10}$(dose) data was fitted to the observed probability of illness using the beta-Poisson model. However, it is noted (Figure A3.1), that the variance in the probability of illness data is lower at low doses and very high doses, but larger in the intermediate range. Accordingly, in a second approach, the $\log_{10}$(dose) data was fitted to the logarithm of the observed probability of illness data to assess the significance of the stochastic assumption on the best-fitting model parameters. The logarithm was chosen as an example of an established variance-stabilizing data transformation.

A further complication in comparison of these models is that at least one of the data sets presented in the Teunis *et al.* (2010) paper was incorrectly transcribed from the original reports. The data from Kasuga *et al.* (2004)[3] for peanut dressing involved an estimated dose of 344 cells, not 3.44 as presented in Teunis *et al.* (2010).

Four models were fitted. The first two used the data as presented in Teunis *et al.* (2010), but with the two variance assumptions described above, while two other models were fitted with the above-mentioned error in the data "corrected" and also using the two, alternative, variance assumptions.

All models were fitted using the Solver routine of Microsoft Excel™, by minimizing the average of the squares of the differences between the predicted probability of infection and observed probability of infection, or the average of the squares of the differences between the logarithm of the predicted probability of infection and the logarithm of the observed probability of infection, as appropriate.

The results are summarized in Table A3.1, showing the fitted parameter values of the four models, the predicted ID50 and the predicted probability of infection for exposure to a single cell.

TABLE A3.1 Data of Teunis *et al.* (2010) fitted to the beta-Poisson dose-response model, using various modelling assumptions

Assumption	Fitted parameters		ID_{50}	$P_{illness}$ from one cell	Mean square error
	alpha	*beta*			
Original data, fitted as $P_{illness}$	5.53	0.121	1 690	1 in 51	0.063
"Corrected" data, fitted as $P_{illness}$	7.83	0.124	2 063	1 in 68	0.064
Original data, fitted as $\log_{10}(P_{illness})$	39.60	0.121	12 256	1 in 333	0.417
"Corrected" data, fitted as $\log_{10}(P_{illness})$	78.86	0.143	9 924	1 in 555	0.387

3 Kasuga, F., Hirota, M., Wada, M., Yunokawa, T., Toyofuku, H., Shibatsuji, M., Michino, H., Kuwasaki, T., Yamamoto, S. & Kumagai, S. 2004. Archiving of food samples from restaurants and caterers—quantitative profiling of outbreaks of foodborne salmonellosis in Japan. *Journal of Food Protection*, 67(9): 2024–2032.

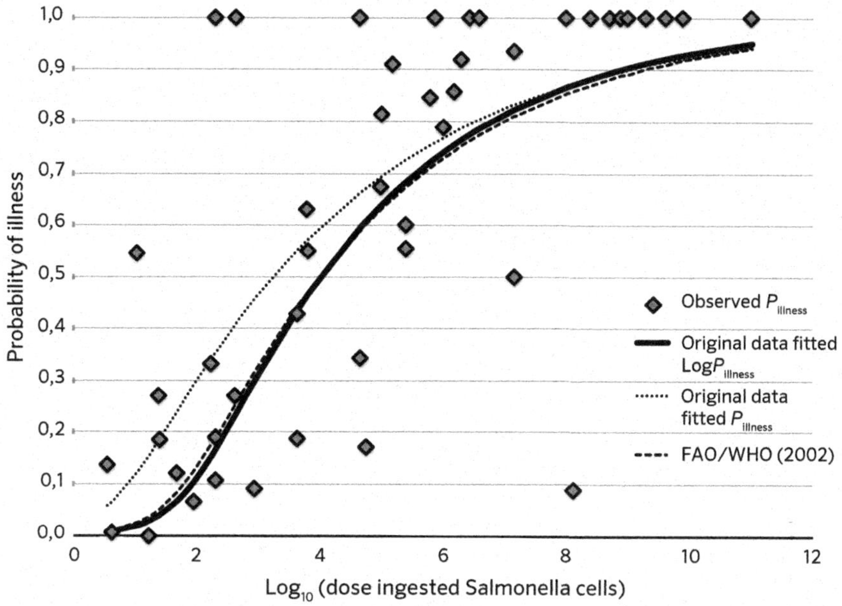

FIGURE A3.1 Comparison of beta-Poisson models fitted, with different variance assumptions, to the data of Teunis et al. (2010) and compared with the FAO/WHO (2002) model

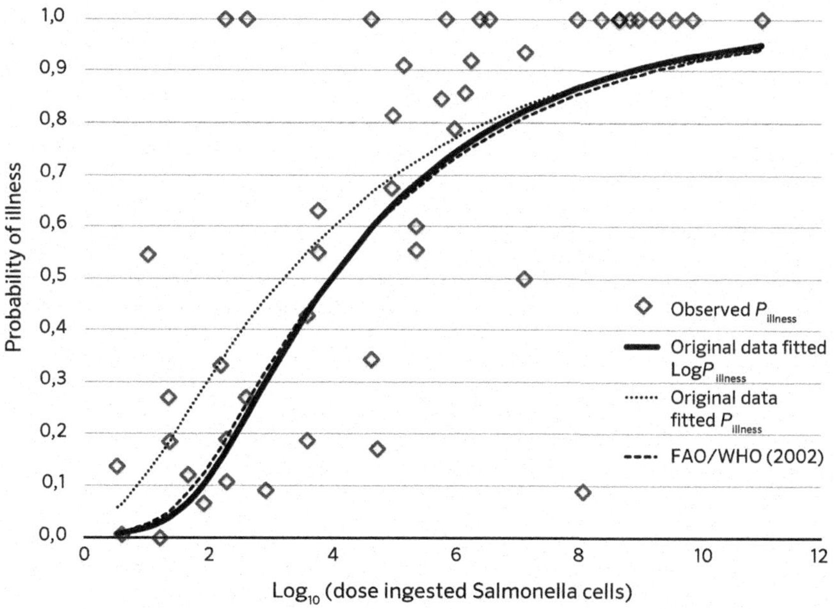

FIGURE A3.2 Comparison of beta-Poisson models fitted, with different variance assumptions and the effect of correcting the transcription error in data, with the data of Teunis *et al.* (2010) and compared with the FAO/WHO (2002) model

Figures A3.1 and A3.2 are presented to further facilitate comparison of these models, at both the ID_{50}, and low dose levels. The figures show that the Teunis *et al.* (2010) data set, when fitted to $\log_{10}(P_{illness})$ data, irrespective of the transcription error, leads to a beta-Poisson model that is very similar to the FAO/WHO (2002) model. The figures also show that correction of the data transcription "error" has very little effect on the fitted model, while the variance assumption has a large effect on both the predicted ID_{50} and predicted probability of illness at low doses.

Based on this analysis, and that in Annex 2, the FAO/WHO (2002) model was selected for the risk assessment calculations in this report.

FAO/WHO Microbiological Risk Assessment Series

1 Risk assessments of *Salmonella* in eggs and broiler chickens: Interpretative Summary, 2002

2 Risk assessments of *Salmonella* in eggs and broiler chickens, 2002

3 Hazard characterization for pathogens in food and water: Guidelines, 2003

4 Risk assessment of *Listeria monocytogenes* in ready-to-eat foods: Interpretative Summary, 2004

5 Risk assessment of *Listeria monocytogenes* in ready-to-eat foods: Technical Report, 2004

6 *Enterobacter sakazakii* and microorganisms in powdered infant formula: Meeting Report, 2004

7 Exposure assessment of microbiological hazards in food: Guidelines, 2008

8 Risk assessment of *Vibrio vulnificus* in raw oysters: Interpretative Summary and Technical Report, 2005

9 Risk assessment of choleragenic *Vibrio cholerae* 01 and 0139 in warm-water shrimp in international trade: Interpretative Summary and Technical Report, 2005

10 *Enterobacter sakazakii* and *Salmonella* in powdered infant formula: Meeting Report, 2006

11 Risk assessment of *Campylobacter* spp. in broiler chickens: Interpretative Summary, 2008

12 Risk assessment of *Campylobacter* spp. in broiler chickens: Technical Report, 2008

13 Viruses in food: Scientific Advice to Support Risk Management Activities: Meeting Report, 2008

14 Microbiological hazards in fresh leafy vegetables and herbs: Meeting Report, 2008

15 *Enterobacter sakazakii* (*Cronobacter* spp.) in powdered follow-up formula: Meeting Report, 2008

16 Risk assessment of *Vibrio parahaemolyticus* in seafood: Interpretative Summary and Technical Report, 2011

17 Risk characterization of microbiological hazards in food: Guidelines, 2009.

18 Enterohaemorragic *Escherichia coli* in meat and meat products: Meeting Report, 2010

19 *Salmonella* and *Campylobacter* in chicken meat: Meeting Report, 2009

20 Risk assessment tools for *Vibrio parahaemolyticus* and *Vibrio vulnificus* associated with seafood: Meeting Report, 2020

21 *Salmonella* spp. In bivalve molluscs: Risk Assessment and Meeting Report, In press

22 Selection and application of methods for the detection and enumeration of human pathogenic *Vibrio* spp. in seafood: Guidance, 2016

23 Multicriteria-based ranking for risk management of food-borne parasites, 2014

24 Statistical aspects of microbiological criteria related to foods: A risk managers guide, 2016

25 Risk-based approach for the control of *Trichinella* in pigs and *Taenia saginata* in beef: Meeting Report, 2020

26 Ranking of low moisture foods in support of microbiological risk management: Meeting Report and Systematic Review, In press

27 Microbiological hazards associated with spices and dried aromatic herbs: Meeting Report, In press

28 Microbial Safety of lipid based ready-to-use foods for the management of moderate acute and severe acute malnutrition: First meeting report, 2016

29 Microbial Safety of lipid based ready-to-use foods for the management of moderate acute and severe acute malnutrition: Second meeting report, 2021

30 Interventions for the Control of Non-typhoidal *Salmonella* spp. in Beef and Pork: Meeting Report and Systematic Review, 2016

31 Shiga toxin-producing *Escherichia coli* (STEC) and food: attribution, characterization, and monitoring, 2018

32 Attributing illness caused by Shiga toxin-producing *Escherichia coli* (STEC) to specific foods, 2019

33 Safety and Quality of Water Used in Food Production and Processing, 2019

34 Foodborne Antimicrobial Resistance: Role of the Environment, Crops and Biocides, 2019.